THE HEALTH CARE MANAGER'S GUIDE TO CONTINUOUS QUALITY IMPROVEMENT

D0939193

**Wendy Leebov, Ed.D., and
Clara Jean Ersoz, M.D.**

Authors Choice Press
New York Lincoln Shanghai

The Health Care Manager's Guide to Continuous Quality Improvement

Authors Choice Press
an imprint of iUniverse, Inc.

For information address:
iUniverse
2021 Pine Lake Road, Suite 100
Lincoln, NE 68512
www.iuniverse.com

Originally published by American Hospital Publishing, Inc.

The views expressed in this publication are strictly those of the authors
and do not necessarily represent official positions of the American Hospital Association.

Cover illustrations by Jean-Francois Podevin. Copyright ©1989 by The Image Bank

ISBN: 0-595-28366-7

Printed in the United States of America

Contents

List of Figures

List of Tables

About the Authors

Wendy Leebov, Ed.D., is currently the associate vice-president of human resources at Albert Einstein Healthcare Foundation in Philadelphia. She was previously the founder and president of The Einstein Consulting Group, a subsidiary of the Albert Einstein Healthcare Foundation. The Einstein Consulting Group helps health care organizations achieve continuous improvement in service and quality. The group's work has been featured in *Newsweek, Healthcare Management Review, The Washington Post, Hospitals, Journal of Healthcare Marketing,* and *Healthcare Marketing Report.*

Dr. Leebov is a nationally recognized author, speaker, workshop leader, and retreat facilitator. Her writings include many articles, training curricula, and the following books: *Health Care Managers in Transition: Shifting Roles and Changing Organizations* (with Gail Scott, M.A., Jossey-Bass, Inc., 1990); *Service Excellence: The Customer Relations Strategy for Health Care* (American Hospital Publishing, 1988); and *Patient Satisfaction: A Guide to Practice Enhancement* (with Michael Vergare, M.D., and Gail Scott, M.A., Medical Economics Books, 1989).

She received her doctorate in human development from the Harvard Graduate School of Education.

Clara Jean Ersoz, M.D., M.S.H.A., is vice-president, medical affairs, at St. Clair Memorial Hospital in Pittsburgh. Dr. Ersoz has served on the clinical faculty for the Joint Commission on Accreditation of Healthcare Organizations, for which she taught advanced strategies for medical staff leadership. She is clinical assistant professor of anesthesia and critical care medicine at the University of Pittsburgh. She is a diplomate of both the American Board of Anesthesiology and the American Board of Medical Management.

Dr. Ersoz is a graduate of Chatham College and received her medical degree from the University of Pittsburgh Medical School. She took residency training at Shadyside Hospital in Pittsburgh, the University of Toronto in Canada, Mercy Hospital in Pittsburgh, and the University of Pittsburgh. In addition to her medical degree, Dr. Ersoz holds a master of science in health administration from the University of Colorado.

Preface

Health care organizations are increasingly embracing continuous quality improvement as an essential objective for every level of employee and every physician. Although conferences, workshops, books, and articles abound to help health care executives develop or strengthen their organization's overall approach to quality improvement, relatively little information is available for managers who, at every level, must translate the principles of continuous improvement into practical reality.

To benefit their organizations, managers must incorporate into their daily work a system for continuous improvement. This means focusing attention, time, and effort on meeting internal and external customer expectations. It also means knowing who your customers are, tuning into their needs and expectations, establishing processes for soliciting customer feedback, developing indicators, monitoring operational performance and then using this information to plan and execute effective, corrective action in a timely fashion.

Designed for department directors, physician chiefs, product line managers, improvement team leaders and facilitators, administrators, and committee chairpeople, this book is a practical guide to managing for continuous improvement. It is not designed to help health care executives plan comprehensive, organizationwide total quality improvement strategies. Nor is it a comprehensive guide to facilitating improvement teams. Rather, it is intended to help managers, especially middle managers and physician chiefs of staff, make customer-driven management and continuous improvement an everyday routine.

Part I introduces the concept of continuous quality improvement. Chapter 1 defines quality in health care and identifies opportunities for integrating traditional quality assurance models with continuous improvement models. Chapter 2 presents an overview of customer-driven management and the health care manager's role in continuous improvement and provides two self-assessment tests to help readers gauge their mind-set and skills with regard to quality management.

Part II explores customer-driven management and process improvement—two models that build data-driven self-correction into your daily management routine. Each step in these processes is explained, and practical aids are provided for starting up these processes within your realm of influence, including suggested approaches to making each step operational. Chapter 3 presents an overview of the customer-driven management process.

Chapter 4 explores how to identify your customers and their expectations and the professional standards that are key to quality. Chapter 5 describes how to translate customer expectations and professional standards into process or operational requirements. Chapter 6 examines measurement methods and explains how to incorporate a measurement system to track performance related to customer expectations and professional standards. Chapter 7 explores ways to understand and translate the data into improvement priorities and corrective action. Chapter 8 describes the pivotal process improvement model and how to use this model to pursue and make improvements.

Part III provides an in-depth discussion of the most useful and user-friendly tools of process improvement—tools that make processes, root causes of problems, decisions, and plans *visible* and therefore easy to understand, discuss, and manipulate.

Resources on quality improvement are plentiful, particularly those that address the tools of quality improvement. This book is less exhaustive and, we hope, less exhausting. We focus on a select group of tools that we and many health care managers have found to be the easiest and most helpful tools that require no statistical know-how. Because practice is required to become adept at their use, we believe you will achieve greater results by learning these versatile tools well, rather than using a larger variety of tools without having had the chance to achieve mastery and confidence in their use.

The tools presented in this text are applied to health care situations. You are shown how to use them in your department as well as with multidisciplinary or cross-functional teams to take advantage of improvement opportunities with efficiency and effectiveness. The text describes the purposes of each tool, discusses how and when to use it, and presents real-life examples of its use in health care organizations.

The tools for collecting and displaying data are presented in chapter 10. They are:

- Focus groups
- Surveys
- Check sheets
- Logs
- Histograms
- Pareto charts
- Trend charts, run charts, and control charts

The tools for identifying improvement opportunities and pursuing them are described in chapter 11; these are the tools for organizing your thinking, making quality decisions, planning for effective implementation, and communicating your process and results. They are:

- Flowcharts
- Brainstorming
- Affinity charts
- Relationship diagrams
- Cause-and-effect diagrams
- Force-field analyses
- Decision matrices
- Tree diagrams
- Action planning

Part IV addresses the concerns many managers have expressed about making changes in the directions proposed. Chapter 12 highlights the opportunities available to make your organization better, to engage and stimulate your staff in the pursuit of continuous improvement, and through the process, to reap significant benefits for your customers, your staff, and yourself as a thriving, learning, effective professional. Chapter 13 provides an example of process improvement that shows how the tools of continuous improvement can be integrated and used to improve health care processes.

Finally, the appendix provides a list of excellent resources you can use to learn more about the process of continuous quality improvement.

We hope this book is helpful to you in building the skills and attitudes necessary to facilitate continuous improvement with your staff and teams. We also hope it is helpful in building the confidence and optimism needed to tackle long-standing frustrations, inefficiencies, and problems in ways that generate experiments, solutions, improvements, and even breakthroughs.

Acknowledgments

The authors wish to thank the many people who contributed to the substance and production of this book:

- The talented managers, staff, and physicians of St. Clair Hospital in Pittsburgh, who are pioneers in health care quality improvement and whose questions, insights, and collaboration have helped us translate theory into practice.
- The clients of The Einstein Consulting Group, who contributed questions, examples, and insights and helped us to focus on what managers need to do to become active in the quest for continuous improvement.
- Beverly Begovich, Eileen Chisari, Lucy Schoupp, and Beth Stenger of St. Clair Hospital, who supported this effort by contributing valuable models and helping to clarify fuzzy concepts in the gray area between quality assurance and continuous quality improvement.
- Einstein Consulting Group staff members Mary Ellen Kelly, Lori Anderson, Wesley Hilton, Leslie Nickerson, Jackie Reilly, Joan Theetge, Sheila Wallace, Kelly Yeager, and Virginia Yeager for their endless support, patience, and skill and for their commitment to the premise that "quality is in the details."
- Susan Afriat, Jack Fein, Allan Geller, Pat Mathews, Richard Rosen, and Gail Scott, the dedicated and determined team of consultants with The Einstein Consulting Group who helped to develop and demystify key concepts, models, and approaches and who fueled our persistence with their dedication to making health care better.
- Benjamin Snead, president, St. Clair Hospital, who had the vision to begin the Quality Enhancement Strategy (QUEST) at St. Clair Hospital in 1988.
- Martin Goldsmith, Janine Kilty, and Robert Stutz of the Albert Einstein Healthcare Foundation for their enduring guidance and support.
- Leland Kaiser, a teacher and mentor who taught Clara Jean Ersoz systems thinking, inspired her to take a holistic view of the universe, and helped her to understand the concept of systems within systems within systems.
- The pacesetters and teachers in the quality improvement field (W. Edwards Deming, Joseph Juran, Bob King, Don Berwick, Brent James, and many others) who have helped and will continue to help health care professionals translate commitment to quality into effective strategy and action.
- Liz Dunn, Nikki Gollub, and Namik Ersoz, whose support of and patience with our projects are endless.

Part I

Revitalizing Quality Management

Chapter 1

The Shifting Profile of Quality in Health Care

Today's health care organizations are focusing on quality and continuous improvement to an unprecedented degree. Achieving and sustaining a reputation for quality and continuous improvement are both ethical and business necessities in our present health care environment:

- Turbulence and change threaten quality at the very time that consumers, purchasers of health care, and health care professionals are demanding higher levels of quality and service than ever before. The organization that does not focus attention on quality improvement inevitably allows quality to slip, resulting in the dissatisfaction of customers, employees, and physicians alike.
- Quality is the right and ethical thing. We are in the business of caring. Anything less than a demonstrated commitment to high-quality performance by ourselves and our organizations is a disservice to all of our customers—particularly to the patients who place themselves in our hands.
- Quality helps patients achieve optimal health outcomes in an atmosphere of excellent service. When we excel in meeting and exceeding our customers' expectations, our customers spread the good word. Customers value quality and look for the provider who will not only satisfy, but exceed their requirements.
- A commitment to quality reduces expenditures. Research on the cost of quality repeatedly shows that 20 to 30 percent of a typical organization's expenses are the result of redundancy of effort, rework, error, inefficiency, recurrent problems, untrained personnel, and cumbersome systems.
- On the revenue side of the equation, 10 percent in lost revenue is attributable to problems in maintaining quality.
- The organization that eliminates quality problems spares its customers and staff frustration.
- Attention to quality helps health care professionals to feel invested in their work and proud to be associated with their organization. Health care professionals want to be associated with an organization that stands for excellence in all it pursues— one that does not take quality for granted by falling back complacently on "the way we've always done things here." An organization that can honestly boast about

quality and maintain its commitment to continuous improvement will attract and retain talented staff.

- The organization that is focused on quality and that has developed documentable and effective strategies for ensuring continuous quality improvement will more easily meet the standards of outside review organizations such as the Joint Commission on Accreditation of Healthcare Organizations (Joint Commission).

□ Quality

As in other industries, quality in health care means *doing the right things right* and *making continuous improvements.*

Doing the Right Things Right

As the following matrix suggests, your organization and everyone in it can do the right or wrong things and do them in a right or wrong way.

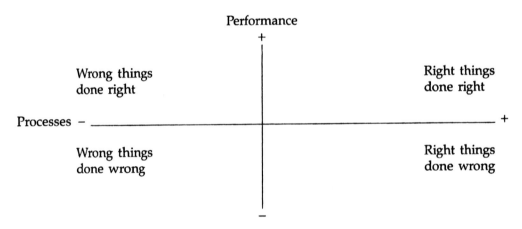

Processes that meet customer expectations in a streamlined, cost-effective manner are the right things. *Performance* by people and departments that conforms to these processes is things done right. Fortunately, processes and performance interact. When you clarify and improve processes, performance improves as a result.

Following are examples of the four possibilities:

1. *Doing the right things wrong.* You have a great piece of equipment that is capable of producing very accurate and important test results, but the technicians don't use the equipment correctly; or your organization has designed a very accessible chart retrieval system, but the people using it don't return borrowed charts.
2. *Doing the wrong things wrong.* You have an inefficient system for scheduling patients for preadmission tests and the people using this system make many mistakes when they enter people's names and appointment times.
3. *Doing the wrong things right.* Using that same inefficient scheduling system, employees do a perfect job of entering people's names, appointment times, and all other information.
4. *Doing the right things right.* You have excellent equipment and you use it correctly 100 percent of the time.

Traditional quality assurance and continuous quality improvement meld at the "right things done right" interface. The emphasis in traditional quality assurance has been on monitoring whether the appropriate things are being done correctly. If they are not, actions are taken to correct *individual performance* to ensure better results in the future. In continuous quality improvement, the emphasis is also on doing the right things right, but in the face of problems, attention is directed first and foremost to the *process*. Improvement efforts focus on identifying the root causes of problems (causes stemming from the process rather than individual performance), intervening to reduce or eliminate these causes, and taking steps to correct the process.

Both process and performance are important when it comes to quality. Processes, policies, and jobs must be designed to reflect the best, most effective methods for getting the job done, to eliminate inefficiencies, and to ensure that quality is built into the way we do things. That means focusing attention on out-of-date systems and processes, replacing old-fashioned methods and obsolete practices with smooth, streamlined, consistently effective methods for getting the appropriate result. Additionally, our people and departments must have the competence to reliably follow our processes and procedures so that the way things are actually done is consistent with those well-conceived designs.

In doing the right things right and making continuous improvements, one should achieve the following:

- Optimal clinical outcomes for patients
- Satisfaction for *all* customers
- Retention of talented staff
- Financial viability

Optimal Clinical Outcomes

Although patients cannot always judge clinical quality, the professionals in your organization can. In the clinical arena, doing the right things right is analogous to *doing appropriate things effectively*. The question to be asked is: Is this action relevant and necessary (appropriate), and, if so, how can we be sure it will be done right (effectively)? The previous matrix is revised as follows to reflect the clinical arena.

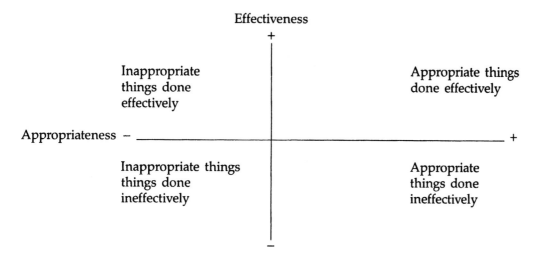

This model is applied in the next few paragraphs to a hypothetical patient hospitalized for a cholecystectomy.

Appropriate things done ineffectively (right things done wrong). A patient appropriate for gallbladder removal sustains a series of preventable complications. For example, the hepatic artery is injured; or the right antibiotic is prescribed at the right dose and for the right time, but it is not delivered or administered on time for prophylactic administration before surgery. It is often easier for patients to perceive things being done wrong than it is for them to see that the wrong things are being done.

Appropriate things done effectively (right things done right). If you were doing the right things right, all care would be appropriate. The patient would meet diagnostic criteria to indicate removal of the gallbladder. If antibiotics were prescribed, the right drug at the right time and in the right dose would be prescribed and administered. There would be no avoidable complications of either the surgery or the process of care. The surgery would be performed expeditiously and skillfully without the development of infection.

Inappropriate things done effectively (wrong things done right). Assume that the patient does not meet clinical criteria for having a cholecystectomy, but the surgeon recommends it and the patient undergoes the procedure. The surgery is inappropriate. All goes well during the surgery, and the patient is discharged in a timely fashion without complications or errors. Being in a position to evaluate outcomes better than appropriateness, the patient believes that the right things were done right. It is up to health care providers to apply their professional standards to ensure that the right things are being done for patients *and* being done right.

Another example of wrong things done right involves the administration of antibiotics for prophylaxis. If the patient doesn't need antibiotic prophylaxis or doesn't need a third-generation cephalosporin for antibiotic prophylaxis and it is administered at the right time and in the right dose, you have another example of doing the wrong things right, or the inappropriate things effectively.

Inappropriate things done ineffectively (wrong things done wrong). Doing inappropriate things ineffectively falls into the ultimate disaster zone. The most obvious example of this situation is that of a patient who dies as the result of undergoing an unnecessary surgical procedure.

The preceding model points out that even if patients perceive health care services to be of high quality, professionals must use their expertise to judge the appropriateness and effectiveness of decisions made on behalf of those patients and the process of care provided. Optimal clinical outcomes will then result.

Satisfaction for All Customers

The use of the broad, inclusive term *customer* helps us to focus improvement on the multiple constituents that are important to a health care organization. Many different groups of customers judge the quality of health care services—patients, their families and friends, physicians, internal customers, payers, and the community. Each of these customer groups has expectations of the organization's service.

For example, most patients want the best state of health they can achieve; convenient, timely service; courteous, compassionate treatment from the staff; and accurate information about their condition. Their families and friends also typically want sufficient information, access to the patient, and responsiveness and compassion from hospital staff members. Physicians want your organization to be user-friendly (easy to practice in) and supportive of their efforts to serve their patients. Payers want information in a timely fashion and optimal health outcomes for patients at the lowest possible cost.

Internal customers (co-workers and other departments) also need to be considered. Every employee and department has other employees and departments as internal customers. If every employee and department had their expectations met by their internal customers, the organization would be an aggravation-free and wonderful place to work.

Customers judge quality by the extent to which you meet these expectations or "requirements." Although some health care professionals find the use of the word *customers* alien when applied to patients and their families, the customer concept is key to determining the right things in our definition of quality as doing the right things right. Patients are customers of health care services in that they choose among and use health care services, and they have certain expectations of these services. When their expectations are not met, the product or service is perceived as lacking in quality. If our services do not meet our customers' criteria for quality, we are doing the wrong things. Customer expectations also help to define objectives for continuous improvement. You select as priorities for improvement those problems or opportunities that help you:

- Sustain your ability to meet customers' expectations consistently
- Meet customers' rising or changing expectations
- Exceed your customers' expectations

For example, one of the pharmacy department's principal customers is the nursing unit. The nurses, in turn, must deliver timely, accurate doses of medication to their customers—the patients. Thus, if the director of the pharmacy manages a medication delivery system whose timing does not meet the needs of the nurses, the nurses are unable to meet the needs and expectations of their patients. This produces a situation in which nurses either do not deliver medication in a timely fashion or develop their own means of getting around the system to ensure that medications are available. For example, the nurse might stockpile a medication or have someone run to the pharmacy (taking the runner away from the nursing unit). In either situation, the cost of doing business is increased, the satisfaction of the nurse is decreased, and the timely delivery of medication to the patient is hampered, as is the patient's satisfaction.

In short, when customers' expectations are not being met, quality suffers. By using the customer concept (applied to both internal and external customers) to guide improvement efforts, you will increasingly do the right things and enhance quality.

Retention of Talented Staff

Another outcome of doing the right things right and making continuous improvements is greater success in attracting and retaining talented employees and physicians. Competent, caring health care professionals want to be associated with an organization that strives for excellence not in rhetoric, but in practice. When physicians and employees contribute to streamlining systems, making the organization and its processes more customer-friendly, relieving turf tensions, and taking ever better care of patients, they feel better about their work and are much more likely to be loyal to the department and/or the organization. An old adage applies here: "Your job is your self-portrait. Autograph it with excellence."

Financial Viability

Doing the right things right also pays off financially. In order to maximize the three components—optimal clinical outcomes, customer satisfaction, and the retention of talented staff—you will need to make improvements that will reduce redundancy in cumbersome work processes, lessen rework due to avoidable errors, and introduce efficiencies in your use of precious financial and human resources. The results will be tremendous reductions in cost. Your bottom line will reflect increases in revenue from boosts in business volume that result when customer satisfaction is high, and the high costs of staff turnover and recruitment will be reduced because of greater job satisfaction. Doing the right things right cuts cost and increases business; the net result is sound financial performance—the key to viability.

Making Continuous Improvements

The health care industry is characterized by change. Our services and techniques are complex and continually changing. The rules of reimbursement are unpredictable and beyond the control of health care organizations. Turnover and evolution within the work force are continuous. The needs of patients and their families change. Regulators' requirements are always changing. And relationships among administrators and physicians, physicians and employees, and the employees themselves are constantly changing.

Some of these changes create obstacles to quality improvement; for example, long-standing turf problems inhibit people from crossing departmental lines to solve quality problems, and strained relationships among administrators and physicians impede a sense of partnership in approaching the challenge of continuous improvement. Other changes make things easier; for example, regulatory requirements and the demands of payers for data regarding quality propel continuous improvement forward, as do rising customer expectations in today's competitive environment. The result is that quality is a moving target. The complacent organization can expect not only a downturn in quality, but also a rapid decline in its competitive position as the organization down the street seizes the quality challenge and strides forward.

Continuous improvement is at the heart of the challenge. Perfection is impossible, but improving things by tackling problem after problem and experimenting with improvement after improvement *is* possible. Continuous improvement is accomplished best by improving the processes by which people work, not just by correcting the shortcomings of the people doing the work. As our industry learns more about how to reap the greatest benefits from continuous improvement initiatives, we are replacing the old belief that quality fails when people do the right things wrong with the new understanding that quality fails more often when people do the wrong things right. Industry experts speculate that as much as 80 percent of an organization's quality problems center on work processes and not people; it is these work processes that should be the primary target of continuous improvement initiatives.

All work processes have built-in limitations. First, any process has limited capability; there are limitations in the results produced, which the process, designed as it is, cannot exceed. Second, every process has built-in variability, which is contributed by differences among customers, staff, environmental conditions, equipment irregularities, and so forth. This variability is unwanted because it makes the outputs of the process unpredictable and inconsistent.

Therefore, the two most fruitful objectives for continuous improvement are:

1. To improve or raise the mean level of outputs of the process by improving its overall capability
2. To reduce and control the variability built into the process in order to achieve the desired outputs consistently and predictably

Figure 1-1 illustrates these objectives. Part A of the figure shows the normal curve of performance for a given process. As just mentioned, two components are involved in making improvements: (1) raising the mean level of performance (part B) and (2) reducing variation around this mean (part C). In the continuous improvement process, both objectives are pursued, as shown over time (from left to right) in part D of the figure. The benefits are higher standards and greater consistency and predictability in the performance of the process, which in turn lead to greater consistency and predictability in achieving the desired results for customers.

☐ Strategies That Advance Continuous Quality Improvement

To achieve continuous attention to quality institutionwide, most health care organizations are implementing far-reaching strategies. The following are a few examples of the components of these strategies:

- *Leadership commitment.* Administrators and managers are educating themselves about quality improvement and exploring roles they can play to drive the organization toward quality.

- *Customer expectations.* Organizations are consulting their customers, both internal and external, to understand their expectations and focus their improvement efforts on customer priorities.
- *Managing for quality.* In many organizations, managers and supervisors are upgrading their skills in quality management so that every department and every service throughout the organization is quality driven and improvement oriented.

Figure 1-1. Graphic Representations from Normal Curve of Performance to Continuous Improvement

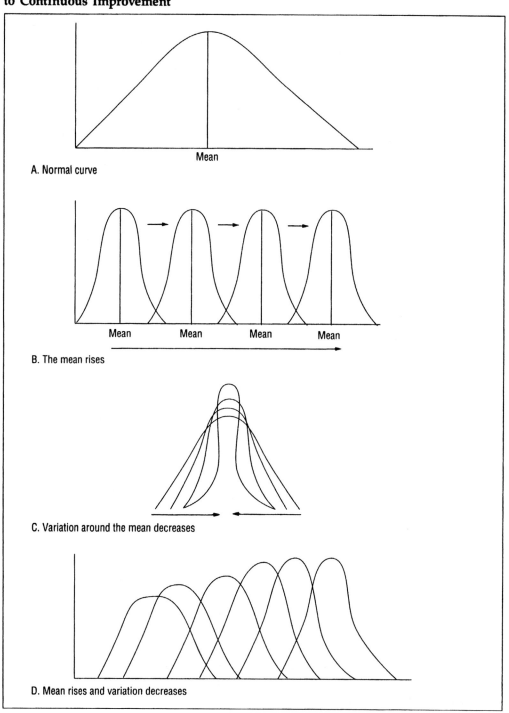

A. Normal curve

B. The mean rises

C. Variation around the mean decreases

D. Mean rises and variation decreases

- *Measurement and feedback.* Because it is difficult to know whether you're winning without a scorecard, many organizations are improving their methods of measuring and monitoring performance related to key clinical and service indicators. Ideally, all health care workers should receive feedback about their own success and their team's degree of success in making quality real on their jobs, within their departments, and in the overall organization.
- *Accountability.* Processes do not work by themselves; people make quality happen. Therefore, people throughout the organization must be held accountable and responsible for doing the things we deem to be the right things—conforming to quality processes consistently and reliably. Many organizations are improving job descriptions, performance appraisal systems, coaching techniques, and other personnel practices in order to improve responsibility for quality performance.
- *Problem solving, process improvement, and prevention.* In most health care organizations, there is so much going on that snags, hassles, frustrations, and waste are inevitable. Organizations are forming teams to tackle problems at their roots and redesign the way work is performed so that problems that frustrate employees, physicians, and patients and unnecessarily consume precious resources can be avoided. This means streamlining systems, creating as much efficiency as possible, and making your organization customer-friendly and employee-friendly, as well as cost-effective.
- *Employee involvement and empowerment.* To advance quality and make everyday improvements, quality-driven organizations involve everyone in the process. To accomplish this involvement, staff members need to be empowered to act, initiate, and affect the system on behalf of their customers, with skill and sensitivity.
- *Staff development and training.* Quality performance requires *skills.* Organizations involved in quality improvement step up their training programs for employees and physicians so that staff members throughout the organization will have the improved skills to do both the technical and nontechnical aspects of their jobs and will become more effective problem solvers and innovators.
- *Communication and teamwork.* Quality improvement strategies fall apart unless the people in the organization function as a well-oiled machine. This takes a great deal of cooperation and teamwork. Organizations are focusing their attention on improving communication and building stronger bridges between individuals, both within departments and across departmental lines. An organization with turf problems will have difficulty in quality improvement because so many quality problems fall into the cracks between departments.
- *Recognition and incentives.* Organizations are reexamining their methods of rewarding people individually and in teams. Rewards and recognition should be linked to meeting quality targets and suggesting and making improvements.
- *Resources allocated to quality.* Serious quality improvement strategies take time and money at the outset. Your organization may have to make a financial investment in quality improvement even though the economic environment is tight. However, the process improvements that result from such a commitment will save your organization substantial time and money in the long run.

The four facets of a comprehensive strategy for continuous quality improvement are displayed in figure 1-2 and further described as follows:

- *Customers.* At the heart of the strategy are the customers whose expectations drive improvement efforts.
- *Performance improvement.* The job of employees and physicians is to competently, compassionately, and professionally serve their patients and other customers. An effective quality improvement strategy focuses on continuously raising performance standards and increasing the consistency of conformance to these standards by people and departments.

Figure 1-2. Four Facets of Continuous Quality Improvement

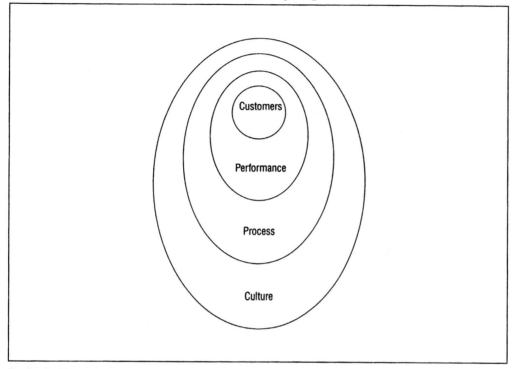

- *Process improvement.* To support your staff and customers, you need hassle-free, streamlined, cost-effective work processes and systems. The effective quality improvement strategy helps people take initiative, experiment, and use state-of-the-art tools to improve processes within and across departments to create a "seamless" organization.
- *A culture that supports continuous improvement.* The effective quality improvement strategy also achieves cultural change by modifying cultural practices (for example, measurement and feedback, communication, reward and recognition, training, and so forth) so that they encourage and support continuous improvement.

Quality and continuous improvement must be an *integral* part of the job of everyone in the organization, and it is the organization's responsibility to focus its members in that direction. No short-term or quick-fix approach is sufficient to make quality and continuous improvement happen. The organizational pioneers of quality improvement have shown that it takes between 5 and 10 years to achieve breakthroughs in quality and to build continuous improvement into an organization's culture. Thus, strategies must be long-term and enduring. To quote John Guaspari, an expert on quality:[1]

> Make no mistake: realizing significant improvements . . . is hard, hard work involving a serious amount of grunting and sweating and heavy lifting on the part of all. . . . It will mean "doing things better", but it will also mean "doing things differently"– which is to say, it will mean change.

☐ Continuous Quality Improvement versus Traditional Quality Assurance

In health care, continuous quality improvement represents a paradigmatic shift when compared to traditional quality assurance (QA). Although health care professionals have always cared about delivering high-quality patient care and have been intrinsically motivated to achieve it, QA functions have been largely influenced and shaped by accreditation requirements dictated by regulators. Specifically, we have done what we needed to do to pass the test of scrutiny by the Joint Commission. Health care organizations focusing on continuous quality improvement are motivated to meet regulatory expectations, but they are also driven to meet the expectations and requirements of all their customers. Their goal is to advance quality in order to provide high-quality patient care as well as to compete effectively and excel, not just to meet regulatory expectations. In other words, the traditional QA function appears to be defensive and reactive, whereas the continuous quality improvement approach is proactive and deliberate.

Different Methods

The means and methods typical of the two approaches are different. In a traditional approach to quality assurance, health care organizations measure performance against standards. They install methods to inspect performance and repair or correct performance that is below standard. With a focus on continuous improvement, prevention—not inspection—is the primary method used. Even when performance meets national and local norms, the organization strives to improve its performance anyway, driven by a "good enough never is" mentality.

The focus in traditional quality assurance is on identifying outliers or "bad apples" and taking steps to improve their performance so that they meet the standard. People and departments with clinical responsibilities are most heavily involved. In a continuous improvement focus, attention is directed not only to special causes of low performance by low-performing people and departments, but substantial energy and resources are also directed to identifying and acting on the so-called common causes of the current performance level. If attacked, these causes would improve everyone's level of performance. The focus is on improving processes and reducing variation so that performance increases for all practitioners, not just those at the low end of the performance spectrum. Also, people and departments with clinical *and* nonclinical responsibilities are involved. In addition to clinical outcomes, efficiency, cost containment, elimination of rework and waste, interpersonal behavior, and the quality of the environment all present opportunities for improvement.

Different Scope

The scope of the two approaches also differs. Traditional quality assurance has been primarily focused on selected departments and elements of quality within those departments. The focus of continuous improvement is organizationwide; it is essential both within clinical departments and across functions to create a seamless organization in which patients, information, supplies, and communication flow, efficiently and without barriers, across department lines. Some of the main differences are summarized in table 1-1.

As health care organizations learn about and embrace a continuous improvement focus, QA functions are rapidly changing to fit this new paradigm. The Joint Commission is gradually modifying its guidelines to encourage health care organizations to focus increasingly on work processes and thus reduce the dissonance between the "old" and the "new" approaches. Also, QA professionals are proving to be invaluable resources, leaders, and internal consultants in helping their organizations to move from a traditional QA function to an all-out, organizationwide drive to improve quality, whether there are glaring problems or not.

Table 1-1. Differences between Traditional Quality Assurance and Continuous Quality Improvement

	Quality Assurance	Continuous Improvement
Motivation	Accreditation	Excel; compete effectively
	Regulator as customer	Heighten satisfaction of multiple internal/external customers
Attitude	Required; defensive	Chosen; proactive
Means	Meet standards	Get ever better
	Inspect and repair	Prevention
Focus	Bad apples; outliers	Common and special causes
	Clinical outcomes	Processes
Scope	Selected departments	Organizationwide
	Within functions	Within and across functions

Reprinted, with permission, from the Einstein Consulting Group, Philadelphia, 1990.

☐ Conclusion

In conclusion, quality and ongoing attention to continuous quality improvement are never accidental. They are always the result of deliberate effort—a matter of strategy. In health care especially, there is so much to do for the sake of our customers that management practices, employee involvement, and organizational culture all need to change in order to meet the quality challenge.

Reference

1. Guaspari, J. The role of human resources in selling quality improvement to employees. *Management Review* 76:24, Mar. 1987.

Chapter 2
The Quality Manager

Improvement in quality results from deliberate effort—effort that managers at every level must initiate and sustain. Although certain dimensions of your role may vary according to the level of your organization's involvement in quality improvement, you should be implementing quality management practices in your own area and in interactions with your staff and customers. If your institution is not yet involved in an organizationwide quality improvement strategy, do not wait. Educate yourself about quality management and begin to apply what you learn. You will gain invaluable experience, enjoy the benefits of continuous improvement, revitalize your staff, and, in so doing, become an indispensable resource to others in your organization once they embark on the quality quest.

☐ The Principles of Quality Management

The manager (hereafter referred to as the *quality manager*) who spearheads and sustains continuous quality improvement fulfills a variety of roles that stretch beyond the traditional concept of management as planning, directing, measuring, and controlling. In his powerful and renowned Fourteen Points, W. Edwards Deming describes the underpinnings of quality management.[1] His principles are summarized below and are the basis of the specific management roles described in later sections of this chapter:

1. *Create constancy of purpose for the improvement of product and service.* Allocate time and resources to continuous improvement with an eye toward serving long-range objectives. In health care, this runs counter to the constant fire fighting and shifting of priorities that have blocked, weakened, and, in many cases, destroyed well-intentioned organizational change strategies.
2. *Adopt the new philosophy.* Deming describes the need for "radical rethink," for deep and fundamental change in which the manager no longer tolerates long-accepted standards, delays, and other impediments to optimal performance and business success.
3. *Cease dependence on mass inspection.* According to Deming, the quality manager rebuilds services so that quality is built into the design consistently in the first

place and not inspected, caught, and fixed at a later stage. It is this principle that is causing health care professionals to question approaches to quality assurance that have traditionally focused on inspecting performance after the fact and then initiating improvement efforts rather than encouraging prevention at the beginning of the process.

4. *End the practice of awarding business on price tag alone.* This means installing measures of quality, not just cost, and taking a broader, longer-term view of cost, which is positively affected by quality improvements.

5. *Improve constantly and forever the system of production and service.* Quality managers hold a "good enough never is" attitude. They persistently hunt for problems to solve and improvements to make; they do not "hope for the best" or "let things ride."

6. *Institute training and retraining.* Quality managers recognize that doing the job right requires training, and, because materials, methods, service, and equipment constantly change, training must be ongoing in order to equip personnel to "do the changing job right." Also, quality managers recognize that training is an investment, not a cost, and they invest in continuous improvement and employee retention by training their staff to become agents of improvement, not just "hired hands" but also "hired heads."

7. *Institute leadership.* Quality managers set their staff's sights on quality, not numbers. Quality managers run interference, remove barriers, and coach staff so they can succeed in doing the job in a way that works for the customer and gratifies the person doing it.

8. *Drive out fear.* This point is pivotal and a real challenge to health care managers schooled in a directing and controlling approach to management. Quality managers invite, model, and pave the way for effective two-way communication and feedback. They know that working in fear is incompatible with cooperation and risk taking. Staff who are afraid do not speak up; they try to hide behind meeting the letter of the law in their jobs, even when they know full well that they are being pushed to do the wrong things. Quality managers recognize the paralyzing power of fear and take steps to build trust, open communication, and adopt a cooperative, experimental spirit with staff and co-workers.

9. *Break down barriers between staff areas.* Quality managers recognize the walls that turf lines and territoriality create and the problems that never get solved because of them. They take steps to ensure that they and their staff understand other people's challenges and difficulties and actively build cooperative relationships.

10. *Eliminate slogans, exhortations, and targets for the work force.* Quality managers do not manage with slogans and hype because they know that employees are rarely the cause of quality problems. They focus, instead, on improving processes and systems so that better performance results.

11. *Eliminate numerical quotas.* Quality managers avoid setting quotas and acceptable levels because these foster complacency and work against driving quality ever upward.

12. *Remove barriers to pride in work.* This, too, requires attention to continuous improvement because people feel no pride in doing a job less well than they know is possible or doing a job a certain way because that way is rewarded by the powers that be.

13. *Institute a vigorous program of education.* Making a point that is different from points about the importance of training, Deming emphasizes that quality managers model continuous learning and self-improvement and encourage this among their staff. They recognize the power of knowledge and broadening the potential of the organization by broadening the potential of its people.

14. *Take action to accomplish the transformation.* Quality managers do not stop at rhetoric about commitment. They know the actions involved in managing for continuous improvement and they build these actions into their routines.

The Joiner Triangle (Joiner Associates) shows the essence of these 14 points in the following simple model:[2]

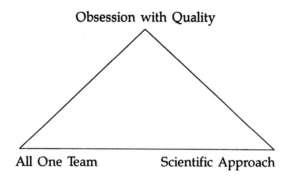

Obsession with Quality

All One Team   Scientific Approach

Although the word *obsession* may appear to be too strong, Joiner uses it to emphasize that managers need to recognize quality as their primary and most profound priority. Joiner shows that total teamwork and a scientific management approach interact to achieve all-encompassing quality. The *scientific approach* involves managing not by instinct or intuition, but by systematically seeking meaningful information and using it to make informed decisions. It involves understanding the nature of variation and the critical importance of reducing variation in order to achieve predictable, consistent, and dependable quality. Finally, to use a musical metaphor, *all one team*, or wholehearted teamwork, involves not only singing one tune but also playing in orchestrated harmony.

☐ Key Roles of the Quality Manager

The following are the roles that translate a quality philosophy and commitment into quality management. The quality manager should exhibit and strive to strengthen each role:

- *Customer advocate.* Quality managers demonstrate an unflinching determination to satisfy customers. They seek out customers, listen to them, take their expectations to heart, and orient processes and people to satisfy their expectations.
- *Mobilizer.* Quality managers act in accordance with their clear and powerful vision because they abhor double standards. Through communication and role modeling, they make their vision and commitment contagious, helping others to share in it with vigor and resolution. They know that, as John Naisbitt says, "Ordinary people are dying to make a commitment,"[3] and they invite that commitment genuinely and often.
- *Standard pusher.* Quality managers ensure that performance of key processes is monitored. They hold themselves and others accountable for doing the right things right. They proactively seek to improve work processes in order to propel the standards ever upward.
- *Change maker.* Quality managers instigate, welcome, and embrace change. They translate their can-do attitude into pursuing and achieving tangible improvements in processes, the team, and themselves. They experiment and innovate with a spirit of curiosity and adventure, enticing others to join in.
- *Partner.* Quality managers share control with others, which often means giving control away. They agree with Teddy Roosevelt that "the best executive is the one

who has sense enough to pick good people . . . and self-restraint enough to keep from meddling . . ."[4] They value and strive to build true collaboration and partnerships with staff and suppliers. They relentlessly provide effective opportunities for involvement and engagement in important plans, processes, decisions, and rewards.

- *Designer.* Quality managers view themselves not as custodians of the status quo, but rather as architects of new and better ways. They use analytical, listening, and observational skills to understand the way things are being done and use analytical and design skills to revamp these ways in order to achieve better results.
- *Facilitator.* Quality managers know how to facilitate team building, team problem solving, and team decision making. They can run energizing, productive meetings that respect people's valuable time. And they understand and can manage group dynamics so that teams, groups, and committees benefit from widespread participation, the diverse talents of group members, and the ability to reach consensus and make quality decisions efficiently.
- *Overcommunicator.* To describe this role simply as *communicator* is to understate it. To engage others in continuous improvement, quality managers listen, listen, and listen again to customers, suppliers, and staff. They share any and all information that affects people's motivation, performance, quickness to act, involvement, commitment, and ability to contribute value to the organization. They proactively share information about mission, vision, values, goals, progress, problems, trends, the competition, financial performance, costs, experiments, successes and failures, morale, and so forth.
- *Stabilizing force.* Although quality managers push for change, they also install and maintain technically sound, reliable methods for controlling and reducing variation in processes and outputs. Managers can accomplish this to a significant degree with firsthand knowledge resulting from experience, observation, and consultation with customers and staff, but they also learn and apply useful statistical techniques to identify degrees and sources of process variation.
- *Team builder and integrator.* Synergy, or the "whole as greater than the sum of its parts," is what the quality manager engenders through recognition of and assistance in blending the talents of staff, suppliers, and customers. Quality managers value team power: They help people bond with one another and align with a shared vision, and they provide experiences that foster true collaboration among staff and with people in other departments. They use their influence and resources to recognize and reward team cooperation, effort, and results more than individual prowess, achievement, and competitiveness.

The *Wizard of Oz* provides a powerful metaphor for the key attributes of the quality manager. Remember the Tin Man, the Scarecrow, and the Cowardly Lion? The Tin Man sought a heart, the Scarecrow yearned for a brain, and the Cowardly Lion quested for courage. All in all, these three highly prized attributes are key to quality management—brains, heart, and the courage to use them to their fullest for the sake of quality.

If any of the key roles inherent in quality management are new to you, the following steps will help you embrace them:

1. Educate yourself. Read, attend conferences, talk with people experienced in quality management, listen to tapes, make site visits—all to learn about the cutting edge of quality management and avoid what might otherwise be missteps difficult to undo.
2. Clarify your vision of quality and your own personal commitment to continuous improvement.
3. Articulate your vision to staff, suppliers, and customers.

4. Educate your staff about what it means to demonstrate a customer orientation and to strive for quality and continuous improvement, including the key concepts, attitudes, and tactics involved.

5. Engage your employees in identifying customers and their expectations, suppliers and their requirements of them, and the current processes that transform inputs from suppliers into outputs that meet customer expectations.

6. Install and sustain ongoing methods of monitoring and providing feedback on the performance of processes and people so that successes can be celebrated and problems identified.

7. Identify improvement opportunities in current processes and begin to pursue them by involving your staff; learn to follow a straightforward and rational process of planning, doing, checking, and acting (PDCA). (The PDCA model is introduced on the next page and described in detail in chapter 8.)

8. Train and coach your staff to perform the work in accordance with your (and their) best-designed processes; stay close to the action, remove barriers, and provide the resources needed to enable staff to do the right things right.

9. Institute methods for tracking progress and results and recognizing individuals and teams who contribute sweat and ideas in positive directions.

10. *Persist* in the long-term pursuit of continuous improvement. Don't be sidetracked or allow yourself to be consumed by the kind of daily fire fighting that is incompatible with quality management.

☐ Attributes of the Quality Manager

The new job description outlined in the preceding section constitutes a stretch for many managers. In order to grow and change in their roles, quality managers must have the right combination of attitude and abilities, enhanced skills, and the right mind-set.

Attitude and Abilities for Quality Management

The following matrix, reprinted with permission from Jossey-Bass, Inc.,[5] identifies four kinds of managers in relation to this new delineation of what is involved in quality management:

The Willing and Able Matrix

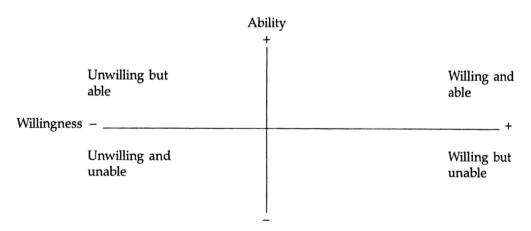

- *Willing and able managers* continuously develop their skills. They have a mind-set that motivates them to sharpen and use those skills in the service of solving real problems and making continuous improvements that result in increased customer satisfaction.

- *Willing but unable managers* lack the ability or persistence to acquire needed skills despite considerable drive to contribute to the organization's quality improvement.
- *Unwilling and unable managers* do not take steps to acquire the skills they need to improve quality. Also, they resist incorporating continuous improvement as an inherent part of their management responsibilities.
- *Able but unwilling managers* have the skills or the potential to learn the skills they need but lack the openness to incorporate these key skills into their everyday actions. Or the culture of the organization deflates their motivation and inclination to use the skills that they have.

Although an individual manager might have a predisposition to fall into one of these categories, the organization's culture also plays a powerful role. By offering high-impact training, mentoring, coaching, peer support, and recognition and rewards in proportion to performance, the organization can help the willing but unable manager to build and apply needed skills. Without these supports, the organization's culture is contributing to skill deficits on the part of its managers. Likewise, organizational cultures that punish managers who experiment and take risks and thus foster an atmosphere of cynicism, traditionalism, and territoriality fuel resistance to change and support "unwillingness" on the part of their managers.

Neither attitude nor ability alone is adequate to meet the challenge of making continuous improvement intrinsic to the way managers do their jobs; both attributes are needed. In addition, leadership is needed along with a culture that supports or even drives managers to achieve new heights of accomplishment, resilience, experimentation, motivation, and learning.

Key Skills for Quality Management

Most able managers already have many skills that are important to customer-driven management and continuous improvement. However, it has become clear from our knowledge of other industries that vast gains can be achieved in customer satisfaction and cost-effectiveness by acquiring additional skills. These skills or tools can expedite and make more effective the application of quality management strategies.

It is important to build into everyday practice an ongoing system for pursuing improvement opportunities and tackling problems. Called the plan, do, check, and act (PDCA) cycle, it is a rational approach to improvement and calls for a repertoire of versatile skills:

- In the *plan* stage, the manager needs to be able to identify customers and their expectations; to describe the current process geared to meeting these expectations; to develop and apply measurement devices that yield baseline data and theories about possible causes of problems; to determine root causes that will, if attacked, result in a more effective process; to generate feasible improvement ideas and select among them; and to develop carefully a plan to implement the proposed improvement on a trial basis.
- In the *do* stage, the manager needs implementation skills so that he or she can effectively institute the improvement according to plan.
- In the *check* stage, the manager needs to be able to monitor implementation steps, performance dynamics, and results so that he or she can draw conclusions about the degree to which the trial-run improvement actually made a positive difference.
- In the *act* stage, the manager needs to have the planning and training skills necessary to develop a plan for integrating process changes into everyday operations so that gains achieved in the short term are held and built into the process from that time on.

The model shown in figure 2-1 graphically illustrates the cyclical flow of these management skills in the rational and systematic pursuit of an improvement. The technology

Figure 2-1. Skills Required for PDCA

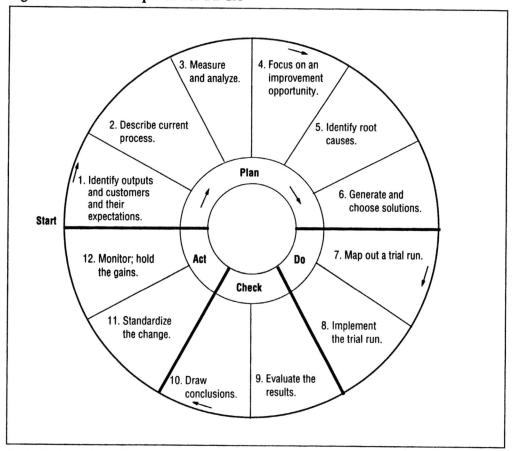

of quality improvement includes many tools that managers and team facilitators can use to help people through this process efficiently so that they can achieve top-notch results. These tools are described in part III of this book.

Your Mind-Set: The Fuel That Drives the Process

Skills and abilities are pivotal and so is your mind-set/willingness. Your mind-set drives your actions. You might be aware of the skills and models that could help you manage for continuous improvement, but if you lack the appropriate mind-set to learn, you will not take the necessary actions or expend the necessary energy. Leebov and Scott[6] describe 10 mind-set shifts essential to managing for improved quality and continuous improvement, as follows:

- From provider orientation to customer orientation
- From tolerance and getting by to continuous improvement
- From director to coach and empowerer
- From employee as resource to employee as customer
- From reactive to proactive
- From tradition and safety to experimentation and risk
- From "busy-ness" to results
- From turf protection to teamwork across lines

- From we–they thinking to organizational perspective
- From cynicism to optimism

More specifically, managers need to understand the following:

- Customer-oriented managers treat customer satisfaction as a much higher priority than what's traditional or convenient for themselves as providers.
- Managers with rising standards believe that "good enough never is."
- Empowering managers increase their own impact by engaging employees in quality improvement and expanding employees' latitude to act to better satisfy customers.
- Managers who treat employees as customers recognize that energized, satisfied employees do not jump ship but, instead, have energy and motivation to contribute to the organization's objectives.
- Proactive managers take the initiative and responsibility to make improvements for internal and external customers and to anticipate and tackle problems before they become fires that must be fought or crises that must be squelched.
- Experimenting managers recognize that you only move forward if you risk trying new ways to make things better.
- Results-oriented managers feel accountable for results and measure their own success by answers, solutions, experiments, and initiatives, not by how swamped or busy they are.
- Team-working managers cross turf lines to confront and solve problems and improve service to customers in an effort to create a seamless organization.
- Managers who think "organization" see resource constraints and improvement priorities from an organizational rather than a self-interested perspective and take the initiative to build a broader stake in organizational improvement among their staff.
- Optimistic managers believe in the possibility of new solutions and even breakthroughs and make their optimism contagious among staff and peers by personally devoting energy to pursuing new possibilities.

In short, today's manager needs not only to manage the status quo, but also to lead the charge of continuous improvement with a mind-set that sparks experimentation, risk taking, and determined persistence. You need to develop and articulate a quality vision, instigate persistently in the direction of continuous improvement, cross turf lines to tackle problems, build effective partnerships with internal customers to expedite needed change, inspire staff to heightened levels of involvement and action, and trigger innovation through risk taking and experimentation. It is a tall order and yet an essential one to quality leadership, a business necessity at every level of management.

☐ Taking Stock: Are Your Mind-Set and Skills Where You Want Them to Be?

To what extent do you have the mind-set and skills necessary for customer-driven management and continuous improvement? Two self-tests are included in this section to help you examine your own tendencies. The first provides a measure of your mind-set and the second a measure of your skills. The scores provide an indication of where you are with regard to these two components and what areas need improvement.

Self-Assessment: Do You Have the Quality Management Mind-Set?

Instructions: Next to each item, place a check in the column reflecting your answer. (Disregard the circles; they will be used for scoring your answers later.)

	Yes	No
1. Do you believe that customers have unrealistic expectations and that you can never really satisfy them?		○
2. Are you and your staff clear about how your internal and external customers define quality?	○	
3. When faced with different ways to do things, do you decide on the basis of what's best for your customers?	○	
4. Do you devote time and energy to collecting feedback from your customers?	○	
5. Are you satisfied with how your department is working as long as you don't hear complaints?		○
6. Do you often communicate a vision of excellence that constitutes a stretch from the way things are currently working?	○	
7. Do you avoid confronting staff even when their performance warrants it?		○
8. Do you communicate ambitious performance expectations to all employees?	○	
9. Do you feel more gratified when you solve problems for your employees than when they solve them without your help?		○
10. Do you feel proud of your employees when they bend the rules creatively to satisfy a customer's need?	○	
11. Do you feel insecure at the thought that your staff can function very well without you?		○
12. Do you see your role as that of coaching, providing tools, and running interference, thereby enabling your employees to serve their customers?	○	
13. Do you balk at employees' requests because you think employees should be grateful for what they already get from work?		○
14. Do you consider your employees as customers whose satisfaction is key to the success of your department?	○	
15. Do you begrudge the time it takes to nurture, recognize, and support employees?		○
16. Do you devote more quality time and energy to the retention of good staff than to the recruitment of new people?	○	
17. When problems arise, do you feel relieved after you've put out the fire and can move on to business as usual?		○
18. Do you usually take on a new project or set a new goal only in response to a request from your boss?		○

(Continued on next page)

(Continued)

	Yes	No
19. Are you a person known for making good things happen?	○	
20. Do you feel too busy to do anything more than handle one crisis after another?		○
21. Do you habitually search for new and better ways within your span of influence?	○	
22. Do you receive new ideas with skepticism rather than enthusiasm?		○
23. Do you deal with mistakes and frustrations as learning experiences?	○	
24. Do you avoid experimenting with new ways for fear of repercussions?		○
25. Do you feel impatient when problems persist over time, and do you want to proceed to solve them?	○	
26. Do you spend a lot of time "trying" and much less time "finishing"?		○
27. Do you track results in order to order to hold yourself accountable?	○	
28. Do you overanalyze a problem instead of moving to solve it?		○
29. Do you take the initiative to seek out other managers to help you with problems or projects?	○	
30. Would other managers characterize you as territorial?		○
31. Do you confront other managers whose actions or inactions have a negative impact on the effectiveness of your department?	○	
32. Are you cynical about solving problems that cut across departmental lines?		○
33. Do you ask your staff for suggestions and ideas about how the organization, not just your department, can be strengthened?	○	
34. Do you withhold information from employees about the organization's status for fear it will dampen their morale?		○
35. Do you accept responsibility for helping staff understand difficult administrative decisions so that they retain their faith in the organization's leadership?	○	
36. Do you find yourself resenting decisions that affect your staff negatively even if you know these decisions are wise for the organization?		○
37. Do you help others see the good in the organization?	○	
38. Are you more likely to complain than to take action to make things better?		○
39. Are you a positive force for change in your organization?	○	
40. Do you see change and experimentation as threats more than as adventures?		○

Scoring: Count the number of checks inside the circles. The highest possible score is 40. The higher your score, the more you already *think* in ways that support the customer-driven process of continuous quality improvement.

Adapted, with permission, from W. Leebov and G. Scott. *Health Care Managers in Transition: Shifting Roles and Changing Organizations,* Jossey-Bass Inc., San Francisco, 1990.

Self-Assessment: Do You Have the Skills Involved in Customer-Driven Management?

Instructions: For each item below, ask yourself the following questions:

- In my span of influence, do I see to it that this is done regularly? Yes or no?
- On a scale from 1 to 4 (1 = low, 4 = high), how effective are my current methods?

	Do I do this? (Yes/No)	My effectiveness (1/2/3/4)
1. I see to it that everyone on our team knows precisely who our internal and external customers are.		
2. I see to it that we consult our customers to identify their expectations by using focus groups, interviews, or other methods.		
3. I have identified reliable measures of the extent to which we meet customer expectations and professional standards.		
4. I translate customer expectations and professional standards into clear operational requirements.		
5. I identify critical control points in our service that influence the effectiveness of the process and customer satisfaction.		
6. I identify and install performance measures at each critical control point.		
7. I see to it that customer satisfaction is monitored regularly using reliable methods.		
8. I see to it that performance at critical control points is monitored regularly using reliable methods.		
9. I make sure performance results are communicated to our staff in a clear, helpful way.		
10. I make sure we communicate performance results to senior management in a way that's useful to them.		
11. I regularly convene staff to interpret our results and decide what to do about them.		
12. When performance improves, I recognize staff for the improvement and help them appreciate a job well done.		
13. Based on our data, I see to it that we prioritize improvement opportunities.		
14. I have in place a reliable and regular system for pursuing improvements.		
15. I use a variety of techniques to involve staff in making improvements.		
16. I follow a rational and systematic approach to making improvements that follows a PDCA cycle.		
17. I use a variety of quality improvement tools to address problems and opportunities for improvement.		
18. I facilitate groups or teams convened for the purpose of making improvements.		
19. I actively analyze work processes, identifying suppliers, inputs, steps in the process, and customers of the process and their expected outputs.		
20. I can name our two current top priorities for improvement and describe a clear approach we are using to pursue them.		

Scoring:

- First, target the actions that you don't currently take. Consider instituting some vehicle for initiating them.
- Second, look at the question of quality. For the actions that you do take, how effective are you? Also, to what extent are you consistently using the skills in your job? Target as opportunities for continuous self-development those skills that you need to strengthen and apply to the job.

☐ Conclusion

As the health care industry embraces quality management, managers are summoned to learn and internalize into routines a demanding and diverse blend of skills and attitudes, some of which reflect radical departures from long-standing management traditions. Although acquiring proficiency in these skills and attitudes requires openness, dedication, and persistence, you are likely to find the learning process and the results of their use both revitalizing and exciting. After all, quality management represents far-reaching opportunities for personal and professional growth and development and increasing indispensability for you in your organization and beyond.

References

1. Deming, W. E. *Out of Crisis*. Cambridge, MA: Massachusetts Institute of Technology, Center for Advanced Engineering Study, 1986.

2. Joiner Associates. *Total Quality Leadership vs. Management by Results*. Madison, WI: Joiner Associates, 1985, p. 5.

3. Naisbitt, J. *Megatrends*. New York City: Warner Books, 1988.

4. Roosevelt, T., as quoted in *Bits and Pieces*. Fairfield, NJ: The Economics Press, 1982, p. 1.

5. Leebov, W., and Scott, G. *Health Care Managers in Transition: Shifting Roles and Changing Organizations*. San Francisco: Jossey-Bass, 1990.

6. Leebov and Scott.

Part II

Implementing Quality Management

Chapter 3

Introduction to Customer-Driven Management

Health care delivery processes are different from manufacturing delivery processes in many ways. One important difference is that the ultimate customer, the patient, receives the "product" as it is being produced with little or no opportunity to inspect it prior to delivery. For this reason, the product must be carefully planned to meet customer expectations and professional standards *before* delivery. Therefore, the model that is presented in this book requires that customer expectations and professional standards be addressed and tested up front.

☐ Specifications for a Management Model

Such a model needs to fulfill the following specifications:

- *Customer expectations and professional standards as a driving force.* Quality management starts with an identification of reasonable, valid customer expectations and professional standards. In order to meet customer expectations and professional standards routinely and focus improvement efforts on high-priority opportunities and problems, your process needs to take its cues from customers whose satisfaction is key to the effectiveness of the particular department and from professionals whose expertise might be needed to define standards on the customer's behalf. For example, outpatients want and expect a short waiting time. Because this expectation is important to them, it makes sense to focus improvement on reducing waiting time.
- *Operations planned to meet customer expectations integrated with professional standards.* Your process needs to translate your customers' expectations and your professional standards into operational requirements. For example, if outpatients do not want long waits for testing, you need to determine what exactly should happen in Outpatient Testing to ensure a shorter wait time and yet still meet professional standards for infection control and proper handling of specimens.
- *Measurement and feedback.* Your process needs to include measures of both process and outcome. You need to develop indicators to determine how well you are

meeting customer expectations and professional standards and share this information with your staff.

- *Identification of improvement priorities.* You need to translate performance data into meaningful information that can be used to identify priorities for improvement. For example, if you survey customers to monitor their satisfaction, you can show trends in satisfaction and focus improvement efforts on slippage or performance below targeted levels.
- *A methodical approach to instituting improvements.* Once you've identified top-priority opportunities for improvement, your process needs to include a thorough and trustworthy approach to designing, implementing, testing, and integrating improvements.
- *Repetition, repetition, repetition.* Your process must be your regular routine so that you are proactive about continuous improvement and not reactive in the face of overt problems or crises.

This process can be illustrated in the approach used by Lee, a hypothetical competitive runner. From benchmarks (other great runners' times), Lee learns what constitutes a "fast time." Lee then determines milestones—how long it should take to get 25, 50, and 75 percent of the way around the track. Then Lee asks a friend to time a run in order to find out actual time versus targeted time around the track. The result is feedback that Lee uses to focus further improvement. Lee then tries to identify the factors causing the gap between desired and actual time and, addressing these root causes, to develop a plan to improve running time by means of speed drills, special speed-training techniques, better nutrition, better shoes, and possibly a different strategy for allocating energy at various phases of the run. Lee then institutes an improvement plan, uses a stopwatch to monitor results, compares them to past results and competitors' results, and creates a new "routine" incorporating the improvement actions that produced a faster running time.

Lee identified a criterion for success, translated it into specific time expectations along the route, measured performance, identified improvement opportunities, instituted experiments to improve performance, and integrated into routine the experiments that paid off in terms of a faster time. This kind of process is intuitive; it comes naturally to some people and not to others. If this kind of process does not come naturally to you, you can learn to institute it step-by-step.

Although there are many models for data-driven continuous improvement, we recommend the customer-driven management process shown in figure 3-1. The first four steps are start-up or planning steps. Once you complete these, you implement the remaining steps in a cyclical fashion, revisiting the start-up steps periodically to modify them in order to embrace changing customer expectations and professional standards.

Ideally, your organization should adopt this or a similar model as the one that all managers use throughout the organization. If people use the same language, the same process steps, and the same data-display devices, they will understand each other, be able to communicate more easily, and build a common pool of experience and expertise as they advance their improvement efforts in the same direction. This alignment across functions and departments will strengthen and clarify the overall system for making continuous improvements happen organizationwide.

☐ Customer-Driven Management: A Continuous Improvement Process

Subsequent chapters describe each step in this model for department management in explicit terms and provide an array of tools you can use to make each step operational. This will help you to start the process, or if you already have a similar process in place, it will help you supplement or continuously improve your current approach.

Figure 3-1. The Customer-Driven Management Model

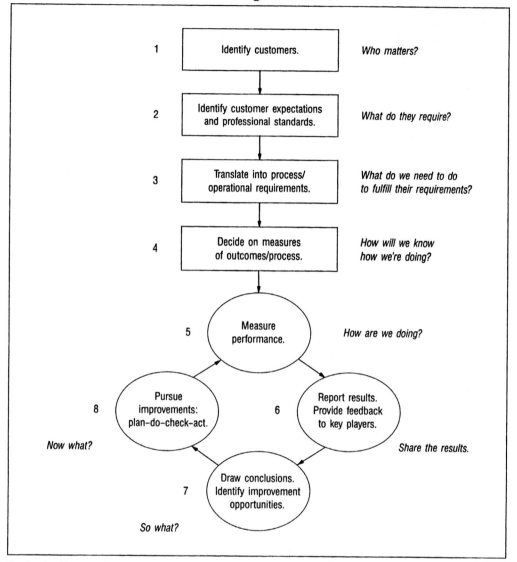

Reprinted, with permission, from the Einstein Consulting Group, Philadelphia, 1990.

Start-up Steps

To launch customer-driven management, you need to make several important start-up decisions. The quality of these decisions will determine how well your department focuses on the most important aspects of your operation. Decisions at this start-up stage address the following questions:

- Who are your customers?
- What are their primary, reasonable, valid expectations?
- What are your professional standards in dealing with these customers?
- What do you need to do operationally to meet your customers' expectations and be aligned with your professional standards?
- What measures or indicators can you use to track performance in relation to operational requirements to meet both customer expectations and professional standards?

Steps 1 through 4, which start the process, are shown in figure 3-1, as follows:

1. Identify customers.
2. Identify customer expectations and professional standards.
3. Translate both customer expectations and professional standards into process/operational requirements.
4. Decide on measures of both outcomes and process.

Although these steps begin the process, you will need to revisit and update them periodically because your department's responsibilities, customer expectations, and professional standards change.

The Cyclical Steps

Once you've made your start-up decisions, you implement them. You initiate a cyclical, closed-loop process for making improvements. The four steps in this closed loop are as follows:

5. Measure performance using the indicators you selected previously.
6. Report the results clearly and share the results with staff and leaders who are in a position to influence them.
7. Engage staff in drawing conclusions from the results, celebrating when the results are good and identifying and prioritizing opportunities for improvement when they aren't where you want them.
8. Pursue specific improvement opportunities by using a rational and efficient PDCA process and appropriate quality tools to yield improved results in the future.

☐ Conclusion

The key to customer-driven management and continuous improvement is to build this never-ending cycle of activities into your management routines and to pursue it relentlessly.

Chapter 4

Identifying Customer Expectations and Professional Standards

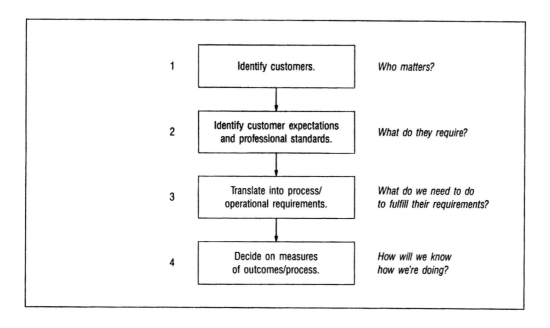

1	Identify customers.	*Who matters?*
2	Identify customer expectations and professional standards.	*What do they require?*
3	Translate into process/ operational requirements.	*What do we need to do to fulfill their requirements?*
4	Decide on measures of outcomes/process.	*How will we know how we're doing?*

Health care organizations and their individual departments must know who their customers are and listen to their customers in order to understand their expectations. Organizations and departments must then tailor their services to meet or exceed the expectations that have been identified to be of greatest importance to their customers.

Many managers believe that their internal quality or professional standards are adequate assurance of customer satisfaction. However, quality standards developed by providers are often designed to reduce inefficiencies or conform to policies rather than to meet customer expectations. Providers' quality standards reflect their perception of quality, which may or may not be the same as their customers' perception. It is even possible for those internal standards to be met despite the customers' perception that quality is slipping.

☐ Obstacles to Meeting Customer Expectations

The following misconceptions about customer expectations can become obstacles to their identification and fulfillment:

We Know What's Important to Our Customers

As health care professionals provide services to their customers and make daily decisions about those services, they commonly assume a certain knowledge of their customers' expectations. Often they think they know their customers' needs and expectations better than they really do.

One of the authors conducted a focus group of former hospital patients to investigate the extent to which satisfaction questionnaires designed by providers contain questions that indeed solicit patient perceptions of what is important to them. At the beginning of the focus group, the following questions were asked: "How do you judge a hospital experience? What characteristics influence whether you would want to use that hospital in the future if you needed further hospitalization?" After people had discussed these questions, the leader distributed copies of the hospital's patient satisfaction questionnaire and asked participants to compare the questions asked on it to their own list of criteria for judging their hospital experience. The result was that they recommended replacing more than half the questions.

The hospital was partly right and partly wrong in the questions it had been asking patients for years. For example, this group of patients said that receiving their meals on time was extremely important to them, but the survey asked only about taste and temperature. Patients also reported that they considered information about their condition and aftercare to be extremely important; yet the survey did not tap patients' perceptions about these critical concerns. As a result of the focus group, the hospital revised its questionnaire to address concerns that were more important to the patients—the patients' criteria for defining quality.

The findings of this focus group were not unique. A discrepancy often exists between what we as providers think customers want and the customers' own expectations.

Our Customers Don't Know Enough about Medical Care to Know What They Should Want or How They Should Judge Us

How many health care consumers can look at an X ray and determine whether it has produced a high-quality image? How many can judge whether their medication dosage is appropriate? Because many of us have technical knowledge that consumers lack, we assume that we are better judges of quality than they are and that our criteria are the right criteria. Although it is important for us to exercise professional judgment and meet our professional standards, this does not mean that our professional criteria are sufficient and the customers' criteria do not warrant attention.

Even in clinical interactions, customers' perceptions are important indicators of quality. Consider the physician who explains a procedure in terms that are medically sound and thorough. That physician's explanation might be professional and accurate, but it may still fail to meet the patient's need, which is understandability. How can the physician possibly judge understandability as well as the patient?

Our Customers' Expectations Change

Customers' expectations change with technology and educational efforts. There is no doubt that the expectations of customers, both internal and external, are a moving target, making the provider's life difficult. But that is no excuse for disregarding those expectations. It just means that you have to consult your customers regularly in order to readjust your understanding of their expectations or renegotiate reasonable expectations with them. When you focus on fixed or static standards, you inevitably miss the mark in terms of meeting your customers' expectations because their expectations are always rising and changing. And because their expectations change, it is that much more important to identify, monitor, and manage expectations, translating them along the way into operational requirements.

Our Customers Make Unreasonable Demands

You might think, "But how can we possibly meet all customer expectations? Customers are increasingly unreasonable!" Although it is true that health care customers are becoming increasingly demanding as providers compete to outdo one another in meeting their rising expectations, customers do not define quality in a vacuum. When their expectations are beyond hope, unreasonable, or even invalid, you can attempt to alter those expectations in order to meet them successfully. You have two options: (1) improve your performance and (2) alter your customers' expectations.

Although patient and physician expectations are largely shaped by your organization's competitors, industry norms, and previous experience with your services, you can still exert considerable influence on those expectations through negotiation and communication. With external customers, you can offer alternatives that address their needs in different ways. You can also communicate about what is and is not possible and why, and then your customers can adjust their expectations accordingly. For example, the health care provider that promises patients that they will be seen within an hour of arrival and keeps that promise achieves much higher levels of customer satisfaction than the one that says it will see all patients within 20 minutes but continues to take 45 minutes. By communicating honestly what you can do and then consistently doing it, you can focus everyday operations and your improvement initiatives on the "valid" requirements of your customers.

It is somewhat easier to negotiate valid or reasonable expectations with internal customers if you are willing to talk with them. For example, in periodic meetings with your internal customers, you can review and discuss their expectations and work to reach an understanding about reasonable goals that you will be able to meet.

☐ Step 1: Identify and Rank Your Customers

Continuous improvement should be driven by customer expectations. Therefore, the first step in installing a system of customer-driven management is to know who your customers are, both internal and external. In this case, *customers* are defined as the people whose satisfaction with your services or products affects your ability to achieve your organization's objectives.

External or *ultimate* customers are people not employed by your organization (patients, their family and friends, managed care buyers, referring physicians, and others) who do business with your organization and who have some choice about where to take their business. *Internal* customers are employees/departments within your organization who contribute to your organization's mission and who depend on your services, products, or "outputs" to serve external customers. You are their *supplier* whether you are supplying patients, information, test results, food, cleaning services, completed paperwork, requisitions, or answers to their questions.

Some departments have external customers as *immediate* customers. For example, nursing and social services serve patients, family members, and physicians directly. Other departments serve external customers indirectly. For example, the storeroom provides supplies to nursing, the emergency department, and the operating suite that are then used by these departments to serve their external customers. Some departments serve both internal and external customers directly.

The same is true for internal customers. They may be your immediate customers, that is, you supply them directly with the outputs of your efforts; or they may be "downstream" or indirect customers. In this case, you do not interact with them directly, but your outputs affect those departments that do interact with them directly and thus have an impact on the external customers as well.

In addition to having customers, every department also has suppliers—other departments or outside vendors who provide them with the "inputs" (people, information, order slips, paperwork, supplies, or the like) that they need to serve their customers. In health care, many departments play dual roles of being one another's suppliers and customers. Although vendors need to address your expectations, you also need to meet certain of their expectations in order for them to accomplish their job. For example, the linen department supplies sheets and towels to nursing (for the sake of patients) and must meet nursing's expectations in terms of the linens' availability, number, and condition. In order for the linen department to meet these expectations, nursing needs to provide clear requests and ample lead time. The supplier–customer relationship is a two-way street in which each party needs to ask, "What do we need to do to make this partnership work?"

According to these definitions, not all health care employees have external customers as *immediate* customers, but everyone does have the external customers as downstream customers whose expectations need to be considered in designing and delivering services. Table 4-1 shows some examples of departments and their customers.

Identify Your Customers

The process of identifying your customers should always involve your staff. By involving your staff in developing a list of your immediate, downstream, and ultimate external customers, you help them see how their contribution fits into the organization's big picture. The process also helps your staff members develop and reinforce their customer focus and think about who they serve instead of what they need from others and invests them as key designers of your department's continuous improvement process.

Table 4-1. Examples of Some Departments and Their Customers

Department	Internal Customers	External Customers
Dietary	Departments who order food for special events	Patients
	Nurses/unit secretaries who communicate about patient food needs	Coffee shop users
		Cafeteria users
Radiology	Nursing Medical records Transportation	Physicians Patients Peer reviewers
Billing	Nursing Information services Admissions Utilization review Medical records Administration	Insurers Patients Physicians Vendors Auditors
Unit secretaries	Nursing Pharmacy Labs Radiology Transportation	Physicians Visitors Patients

There are various ways to develop such a list. One is to brainstorm with your staff about who your customers are. Another, more systematic approach is a simple output analysis in which you examine the key processes within your area of influence and carefully pinpoint their immediate and downstream customers.

An output analysis is done by looking at your function and where it fits into the scheme of things. For example, the following schematic shows your function along with its input and output components:

Supplier———►Input———►*Your function*———►Your output———►Immediate customers ———►Downstream customers

The components are further explained as follows:

- You have suppliers, other vendors and departments who supply you with the inputs (patients, information, or materials) you need to perform your function.
- You receive these inputs and perform certain processes with them.
- When you've finished, you produce an output for either an internal or external customer. This output may be a patient whose treatment is over, a test result, an order that you issue to request a transporter, an entry onto a chart, a charge to be billed, and so forth.
- This output is received firsthand by someone—an immediate customer.
- This output might then be an input to the work of someone else further along the chain of interrelated events involved in health care delivery—your downstream customer.
- Your downstream customer might then serve one or more of the organization's ultimate or external customers.

As an example, these components can be applied to transporters in a hospital, as follows:

- The transporters' suppliers include such departments as admissions, nursing, radiology, physical therapy, and other ancillary departments that issue orders for transport assistance.
- The transporters' inputs are orders for transport services.
- Their process involves pickup, patient assistance, delivery, and the report of job completed.
- Their immediate customers include nursing, radiology, physical therapy, and the patients themselves.
- Their downstream customers can include family members, physicians, and other departments whose work is expedited or delayed by the on-time or late pickup or delivery of patients.

To identify your customers, then, look at your main processes or functions and follow the path of the results or outputs of these processes to their beneficiaries—your customers. It might help to start with the following key questions:

- What are the major outputs of our process?
- What is each service or product we produce?

For each of these outputs or services, determine:

- Who are our immediate customers?
- Who are the customers downstream who have expectations about the quality of our outputs or services?

After addressing these questions, narrow down your list to the key internal and external customers whose satisfaction is most important to the fulfillment of your work group's or department's mission. Figure 4-1 shows how these relationships might be depicted using concentric circles. In the inner circle are the customers directly served by you and in the outer circles are the customers who are in turn affected by the service provided to the inner circle.

Rank Your Customers

Now that you have identified your customers, engage your staff in a discussion of the consequences of both satisfying and not satisfying each customer group's expectations and then rank the customer groups in order of importance. For example, the dietary department has a variety of customers, including inpatients, their family members, out-patients, employees, and physicians. The consequences of disappointing inpatients with poor quality and late delivery of their meals are extreme. Not only do many inpatients need appropriate food in order to regain their strength, but many eagerly anticipate meal-times, expecting at best a taste sensation or at least a respite of comfort that makes their day go faster. When inpatients are satisfied with the food, they are relieved and their family members are appreciative. When they are not satisfied, they, their family members, and often their physicians are annoyed and complain to busy staff. Also, because food quality matters, patients and their families spread the word about the food in your organization as a reflection of your organization's overall service quality. The dietary department's failure to meet food quality expectations costs the organization more when the disappointed customers are inpatients than when other customer groups are disappointed. This is an example of the Pareto principle, which suggests that 20 percent of effort accounts for 80 percent of effect. In other words, satisfying your priority customers can result in a substantial impact on your organization's effectiveness. The chart shown in figure 4-2, or an adaptation thereof, can be used to guide decision making as you seek to rank customers and focus your initial efforts on meeting the expectations of key groups.

Figure 4-1. Concentric Circles Showing Immediate and Downstream Customers

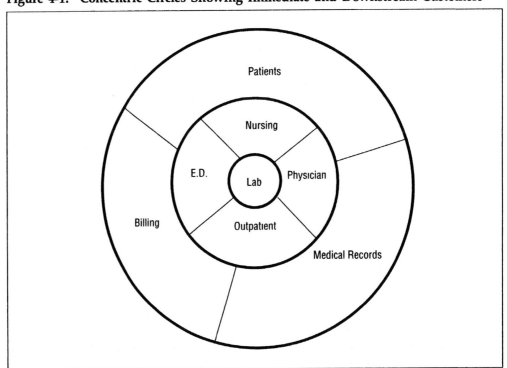

Figure 4-2. Chart for Customer Prioritization*

Customer group	Consequences of satisfying their requirements	Consequences of failing to satisfy their requirements	Rank order (#)

*Discuss your customer groups and the consequences of satisfying or not satisfying each. On the basis of your discussion, rank order these customer groups, with the ones requiring the most quality attention at the top.

Reprinted, with permission, from Clara Jean Ersoz, M.D., St. Clair Hospital, Pittsburgh, 1990.

☐ Step 2: Identify Customer Expectations and Professional Standards

Both customer expectations and professional standards are essential in defining quality and implementing the customer-driven management process.

Identify Customer Expectations

After identifying and prioritizing your customers, the next step is to consult with them in rank order to determine more specifically what they value and what they expect from your service. The challenge is to get specific about their expectations so that you can develop measurable, meaningful indicators. What do your customers care about? Timeliness? Courtesy? Responsiveness? Flexibility? Accessibility? Consistency? Understandability?

In addition to identifying what matters to your customers, you need to establish how your customers rate their expectations in importance. The Attribute Rating Map developed by Marr demonstrates the importance of focusing your improvement efforts on those attributes of greatest importance to your customers (figure 4-3).[1] Once again, the Pareto principle applies. Time, money, and stamina are finite. Therefore, you need to identify the 20 percent of your customers' expectations that account for 80 percent of their satisfaction. This will lead to economy in your efforts and, it is hoped, to a manageable agenda of improvement opportunities. After your customers' expectations or quality criteria are known, you can then identify measures or indicators that will enable you to monitor progress relative to those criteria. Some examples of customer values and their corresponding expectations follow:

- Equipment—that it be fit for use
- Consistency—that no mistakes be made
- Instructions—that they be easy to understand
- Staff support—that it be available
- Paperwork—that it be correct and complete
- Service—that it be prompt

In order to identify the main, measurable characteristics or attributes of quality that matter to your customers, do a needs analysis. This can be accomplished through an analysis of complaints, focus groups, and interviews with customers.

Figure 4-3. Attribute Rating Map: Importance and Effectiveness

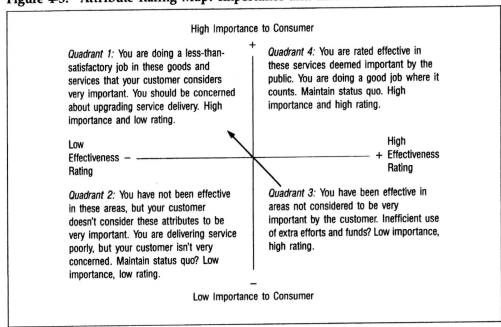

Reprinted, with permission, from *Quality Progress*, American Society for Quality Control, Oct. 1986, pp. 46–49.

Complaint Analysis

Complaints, especially patterns of complaints, are revealing because people generally do not complain unless an expectation of importance to them has been violated. If you can detect the violated expectations underlying complaints, you will have identified a criterion that your customer group uses to judge quality.

For example, consider the maintenance department that tracked telephone complaints about its service. Most people complained about having to wait too long for simple maintenance requests to be processed or having to complete tedious paperwork and wait in line for service, even in an emergency situation. People also complained that maintenance workers would come and go without actually fixing the problem and without explaining when the problem would be fixed. Revealed in these complaints were the following customer expectations: fast turnaround time on simple maintenance requests, a no-fuss process for getting a quick response to stat requests, a problem fixed right the first time, and communication about progress when leaving before the job is completed. All these factors were so important to the maintenance department's customers that they made the effort to complain again and again.

It is likely that your organization already tracks complaints that relate to your department. However, if it does not, you might need to install a system whereby your staff logs all complaints as they are voiced or received so that you can analyze them for quality criteria or customer expectations.

Focus Groups and Interviews

Because focus groups and personal interviews are qualitative and provide rich information, they are especially helpful tools for identifying customer expectations. Focus groups typically consist of 8 to 10 people and last 60 to 75 minutes, enough time for extensive open-ended questioning. The focus group should be led by someone who is able to guide and direct a group discussion effectively without influencing it. Rarely does one focus group provide clear enough direction in any market research effort; therefore, you may need to hold two or three focus groups for more reliable results.

Chapter 10 of this book provides detailed instructions for conducting focus groups. However, the following are the kinds of questions you might consider using in focus groups or face-to-face customer interviews designed to pinpoint customer expectations:

- How would you characterize the service extended to you by this department?
- What do you like about its service? What pleases or impresses you?
- What do you dislike about its service? What irks, frustrates, or disappoints you about it?
- When you interact with this department, what do you look or hope for, for example, timeliness, reliability, courtesy, efficiency? What do you want most from this department?
- In what manner do you want this service delivered?
- If you ran this department and wanted to make its service stand out, what would you focus on? What are the problems? What would you fix? What would you celebrate?
- If you had a magic wand, how would you change this department's people, procedures, services, or systems?

Mapping Customer Expectations

After you have held a number of focus groups in which you have asked your customers to identify their top-priority expectations of your service, present the results to your staff. Then have your staff brainstorm about these customer expectations. Redraw or copy the matrix shown in figure 4-4 and have one person record what people say. The group should then perform the following activities:

- Pick one customer group. Drawing on complaint analysis and/or the focus group results, pool your knowledge of what this customer group wants from your team in terms of service and quality. To prompt your thinking, consider their expectations that fall within each category along the left-hand side of the matrix. See

Figure 4-4. Format for Mapping Customer Expectations

Categories of Customer Expectations	Internal and External Customers			
People skills				
Amenities				
Systems				
Environment				
Technical/clinical competence				
Cost				

whether you can agree on three main expectations or quality criteria. Write these into the boxes relating to that customer group.
- Now, discuss your team's strengths and weaknesses in meeting each customer expectation.
- See whether you can agree on two or three expectations that you want to commit yourselves to improving. Take each of these expectations one at a time, and share ideas for making improvements. Select some ideas and take action!

Go through the same process for each customer group. Use your results to target a small number of improvement objectives. Use the matrix to map out your customers' expectations. For example, a department serving physicians would write "physicians" at the top of one matrix column under "customers." Then, using focus groups, interviews, or other consultations with your physicians, you learn "what physicians expect from us." If they wanted "a timely patient admissions process and fast turnaround of lab results," you would write these expectations into the box where "physicians" and "systems" intersect.

Once you have consulted your customers and identified their expectations, their expectations should be displayed in tables or graphs to help you and your staff focus attention on what matters most to your customers. Tables 4-2 and 4-3 are examples of such tabular displays.

Identify Professional Standards

Customer expectations are essential to defining quality, but customers are not the ultimate and only judges of quality in circumstances that affect people's safety and health. In these situations, professionals must represent the customers' best interests and set professional standards on their behalf.

Professional standards are standards by which professionals perform day-to-day tasks in your organization. These standards can be found in the pertinent professional literature,

Table 4-2. Medical Records Table of Customer Expectations

Key Customers	Features They Want from Medical Records
Physicians	Speedy chart retrieval Sound advice Courtesy from staff
Utilization review	"Partnership" Help in getting needed information
Admissions	Accurate information Complete information Early information Co-worker courtesy
Social services	Timely communication with patients Clear written communication Reliable communication
Our own staff	Working computers Recognition by management Fair expectations regarding work load
Nursing	Speedy chart retrieval Responsiveness to needs Clear requests

Table 4-3. Behaviors of Division of Nursing That Meet Customer Needs and Expectations

Key Customer Groups	Customer Needs/ Expectations	Key Behaviors That Meet Customer Needs/Expectations
RN	Prompt attention	Greet; smile; maintain pleasant and respectful attitude. Be readily available to provide assistance.
	Responsiveness	Ask if assistance is needed. Be flexible to accommodate changing needs.
	Communication	Use direct communication skills: explain, inform, actively seek input. Use problem-solving techniques toward resolution. Provide pertinent patient information in a timely manner. Inform RN if leaving department.
Patients	Prompt attention	Greet in a professional manner. Smile and introduce self. Use patient's preferred name. If unable to provide service/information requested, state "I will get someone to find out for you."
	Reassurance/ emotional support	Touch, smile, listen. Be attentive to patient. Make eye contact; attend in a nonrushed manner. Validate patient's needs, encourage questions. Talk *with* patient/include patient in conversations.
	Communication	Provide information according to skill level and refer to RN as needed.
	Confidentiality	Provide privacy. Discuss patient information on a need-to-know basis. Adhere to patient's bill of rights.
Physicians	Prompt attention	Greet; smile; maintain pleasant, respectful, and professional attitude. Answer phone promptly. Introduce self.
	Communication	Use *direct* communication skills. Explain, inform, actively seek input. Use problem-solving techniques toward resolution. Answer questions according to skill level and refer to RN as needed.
Other departments	Prompt attention	Greet; smile; maintain pleasant and respectful attitude. Answer phone promptly. Introduce self.
	Responsive	Assist, if available. Set priorities according to need.
	Communication	Use *direct* communication skills. Explain, inform, actively seek input. Use problem-solving techniques toward resolution.

Reprinted, with permission, from the Nursing Division of Luther Hospital, Eau Claire, WI, 1990. Developed by Lynn Frank, vice-president, Nursing.

may be developed as a result of government regulations, may result from a need for risk-management practices, or may be found in your organization's policies and procedures.

After clarifying customer expectations, you then need to pinpoint professional standards that are key to effective and appropriate care and service. Step 2 of the Joint Commission's Ten-Step Monitoring and Evaluation Process provides guidance in identifying the scope of care and services for your department/unit.[2] If you are unaware of this, consult your organization's quality assurance specialists. You can also identify the scope of care and services using standard reports available in your hospital, such as case-mix reports, lists of laboratory and medical-imaging tests, lists of commonly used drugs, types of patients using your services, and so on.

Once you identify the scope of care and service, you can develop pertinent professional standards based on this information. For example, if your emergency department receives patients with acute myocardial infarction, the professionals in the department (physicians and nurses) should develop a list of the most important professional standards against which to monitor themselves. These standards might include timeliness of being seen by the physician, timeliness of the administration of thrombolytic therapy, criteria for the appropriate use of thrombolytic therapy, appropriate diagnostic testing, and so forth.

Professionals in your department/unit will be able to identify a host of professional standards that should be met. One of your goals in working with this group will be to have its members decide which are the most important standards to monitor regularly. This decision is often based on volume indicators and standards that deal with care that is either high risk or has high potential for error. Part III of this book presents techniques, such as affinity diagrams and multivoting techniques, that will be helpful in sorting out this material with your staff.

☐ Conclusion

Health care is in transition—from a provider orientation (overattention to requirements defined by professionals) to a customer orientation. It should not be an either-or situation. The challenge is to design requirements that meet customer expectations and also satisfy professional standards developed by health care experts devoted to making decisions that are in the best interest of the patient and the public.

By identifying your most important customers and their expectations as well as the relevant professional standards, as described in this chapter, you will have the information you need to proceed to the next crucial step—translating these expectations and standards into operational requirements. You are on the way to "doing the right things right."

References

1. Marr, J. Letting the customer be the judge of quality. *Quality Progress* 19(10):46–49, Oct. 1986.

2. Joint Commission on Accreditation of Healthcare Organizations. *Accreditation Guidelines.* Chicago: JCAHO, 1990.

Chapter 5

Translating Expectations and Professional Standards into Operational Requirements

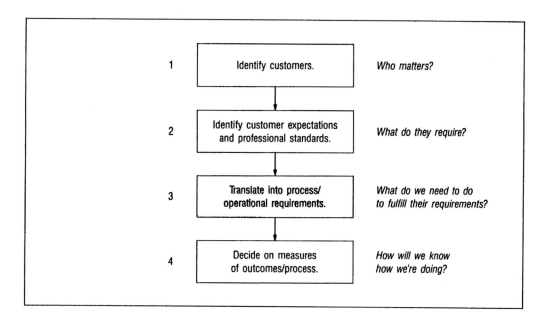

1	Identify customers.	*Who matters?*
2	Identify customer expectations and professional standards.	*What do they require?*
3	Translate into process/ operational requirements.	*What do we need to do to fulfill their requirements?*
4	Decide on measures of outcomes/process.	*How will we know how we're doing?*

After identifying your customers and their primary expectations and clarifying the appropriate professional standards, the next step is to translate these expectations and standards into operational requirements. As a health care professional and expert in your field, you are best equipped to do this. Customers can tell you what they expect and often when their expectations have not been met, but they cannot tell you exactly what to do to fulfill their expectations. For example, most physicians expect speedy chart retrieval, but they could not tell the hospital medical records department what *process* to put into place to make that happen. Professional expertise is needed to design the processes that will effectively and reliably meet customer expectations.

Consider, for example, patients hospitalized for a cholecystectomy (gallbladder removal). When asked to define their expectations, they will most likely cite the following:

a competently performed procedure; a hospital stay during which they are treated with courtesy, care, timeliness, compassion, and respect; and, as a result of the procedure, relief from symptoms. Payers (for example, Medicare, health maintenance organizations, insurance companies) are also customers of this procedure because they pay for it. They also expect a competently performed procedure that involves no complications, a hospital length of stay (LOS) and hospital charges within predetermined limits, and the necessary paperwork and documentation performed accurately, completely, and in a timely fashion.

The hospital needs to meet the expectations of both patients and payers. Although patients can judge the effectiveness of the procedure by their relief from pain (an outcome) and may be the best judges of the service aspects of their hospital experience, they are in no position to judge the appropriateness of the *process* and its many components. Payers, too, can examine indicators of the surgery's success through patient perceptions and such statistics as LOS and costs incurred, but they cannot evaluate the process itself or its various components. The professionals who perform cholecystectomies are the ones who must translate customer expectations into an effective and efficient clinical process.

☐ Step 3: Translate Customer Expectations and Professional Standards into Operational Requirements

Operational requirements are process requirements. They answer the question, "What do we need to *do* to meet customer expectations and professional standards of care?" They include the elements in the chain of activities your department performs that lead to outcomes.

Flowcharts and critical paths are tools that help you translate customer expectations and professional standards into operational requirements. Flowcharts are step-by-step pictures or road maps of processes. They portray sequentially and in picture form every activity or step in a process needed to produce the output that will meet the customer's expectations and professional standards. *Critical paths* are what many clinicians call flowcharts of clinical processes. Reflecting professional standards, these demonstrate how a patient with a particular diagnosis will be moved through the hospital system effectively and efficiently.

The following steps should help in your identification of operational requirements that will meet customer expectations and professional standards:

1. Define the customer expectation or standard as concretely as possible.
2. Examine the steps in your current processes that have a direct impact on meeting that expectation or standard. For example, if the expectation is timely service, list the steps in the process that consume time. If the customer expectation is staff courtesy, list the interaction points or "moments of truth" at which customers will judge courtesy.
3. Sequence these.
4. Then at each point identify quality criteria. What criteria does each step in the process need to meet in order to play its intended part in meeting expectations or standards? If timely service (for example, no more than a 20-minute wait) is the customer's expectation, what is the maximum time this particular step can take? If the expectation is staff courtesy, what behaviors must be exhibited at a particular interaction point for patients to perceive courtesy? (For example, employees must introduce themselves, smile, and say, "Right this way, please, Mrs. Smith.")

Ideally, you should proceed through these steps with the help of employees and physicians involved firsthand in the process. Some managers focus on one customer expectation and standard a month and in their regular staff meetings involve their staff in flowchart-ing and identifying operational requirements related to these expectations or standards. Others convene a small team of people (one knowledgeable about each step in the process) to crystallize the pathway or process critical to producing the output that the customer or standard requires.

For example, if patients coming to your organization for an appointment expect a maximum waiting time of no more than 20 minutes and you can work within that time frame, the outpatient service employees must complete several steps within the 20 minutes in order to meet that expectation. The process needs to be designed so that a defined amount of time is allocated to each of its key steps.

The following diagram shows the situation graphically:

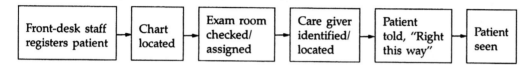

Should the patient be registered within three minutes? The chart located within three minutes? The exam room checked and assigned within three minutes? The care giver identified and located within three minutes? A person found to escort the patient to the exam room within two minutes? Using these time frames, the entire process (albeit some-what cumbersome) would take 15 minutes—a tolerable wait from the patient's perspective.

However, if the patient expectation of a 20-minute waiting time is impossible to meet (that is, you have already streamlined the steps involved in serving patients and your time frame is longer than 20 minutes), you need to negotiate or communicate with the patients/customers to help them accept what is possible and hopefully revise their expec-tation. Then, when you have settled on an expectation you are determined to meet, as shown above, you need to break the process down into its component parts and assign a time frame for each that satisfies the negotiated expectation.

Alliant Health System in Louisville, Kentucky, uses critical paths to translate cus-tomer expectations and professional standards into operational requirements for clinical processes. As mentioned previously, critical paths are flowcharts of clinical processes that staff are supposed to follow in order to serve a patient with a particular diagnosis appropri-ately and effectively. They show the steps in testing, treatment, and follow-up in a coor-dinated, efficient time sequence. Grounded in the experience and expertise of professionals, they specify resources to be used and show how services provided by var-ious departments need to be interrelated and coordinated.

The critical path shown in figure 5-1 demonstrates the process, including the steps, sequence, and timing of services that will produce the best outcomes for patients hospital-ized for diabetic ketoacidosis, while also meeting the expectations of payers. Figure 5-2 on p. 50 shows a flowchart that was developed in response to Pennsylvania state law, which spells out requirements for AIDS testing. The flowchart shows how a hospital translated the "state as customer's" expectations into operational or process requirements.

By defining process or operational requirements, you can ensure that each element in your process is occurring as intended and making its contribution toward meeting both customer expectations and professional standards.

☐ Start with Customer Expectations and Professional Standards, Not with Current Reality

Many organizations or departments set operational requirements that their current process can achieve without strain. The result is that their requirements generally reflect achiev-able performance levels, but only under their current process. Thus, these performance

Figure 5-1. Critical Path for Diabetes Mellitus Ketoacidosis

DIABETES MELLITUS KETOACIDOSIS CRITICAL PATH

Patient Label:

Admit Date: _____   Disch. Date: _____
Expected LOS: 4   Actual LOS: _____
Treatment Date: _____

Methodist Evangelical Hospital:	Path # M0006 DRG 294 (Age > 35)
Methodist Evangelical Hospital:	Path # M0015 DRG 295 (Age < 35)
Norton Hospital:	Path # N0011 DRG 294 (Age > 35)
Norton Hospital:	Path # N0012 DRG 295 (Age < 35)

TREATMENTS/ ASSESSMENTS:	DAY 1	DAY 2	DAY 3	DAY 4	DAY 5 (Discharge)
Consults	Notify: Dietary, Diabetes Nurse Spec.	Dietary completed, DNS completed			
Tests	SMA 6-24, CBC, EKG, U/A, Plasma Acetone, ABG's			Attempt to I.D. precipitating factors; Confirm hydration status (BUN, Hgb & Na); Confirm K+ replacement; Confirm correction acidosis (HCO3); Confirm safe glucose control	
Activity	As ordered/tolerated				
Monitoring	Estb. monitoring plan for Lab glucose, K+, PH; I/O qS; Glucometer q 1-3 hrs × 24 hrs + as ordered/pm	to qid (AC & HS)	D/C		
Medications	Insulin drip × 24-48 hrs (adjust by IV sliding scale; 50cc of Drip thru tubing; 50 units HR, 500cc NS); IVF for hydration; IV K+	Sliding scale Insulin	D/C Insulin drip; Instit. Normal Routine Long/Short Ins.; D/C		

(Each DAY column contains M and U checkboxes.)

Diet	NPO	NPO/Clear Liquids		
Education			Calonc ADA	
			Pt/SO assessm't	Content covered (DKA and sick day rules)
			Reference Manual	Knowledge deficit from assessm't addressed
			Diabetes video	Pt demo understanding
			Give class info & info on outpt FU	Ins. role/dose/time of prevention/Rx for HypoG tm)
				Review Ins. measure & adminis.
				SBGM
				Eval. Diet knowledge
D/C Planning		Initiate Assessm't		Finalize DC plans
				Discharge
VARIANCE ANALYSIS (Comments):				

M = Met (accomplished)   U = Unmet (not accomplished)

Reprinted, with permission, from Ruth Atkins, Alliant Health System, Louisville, 1990.

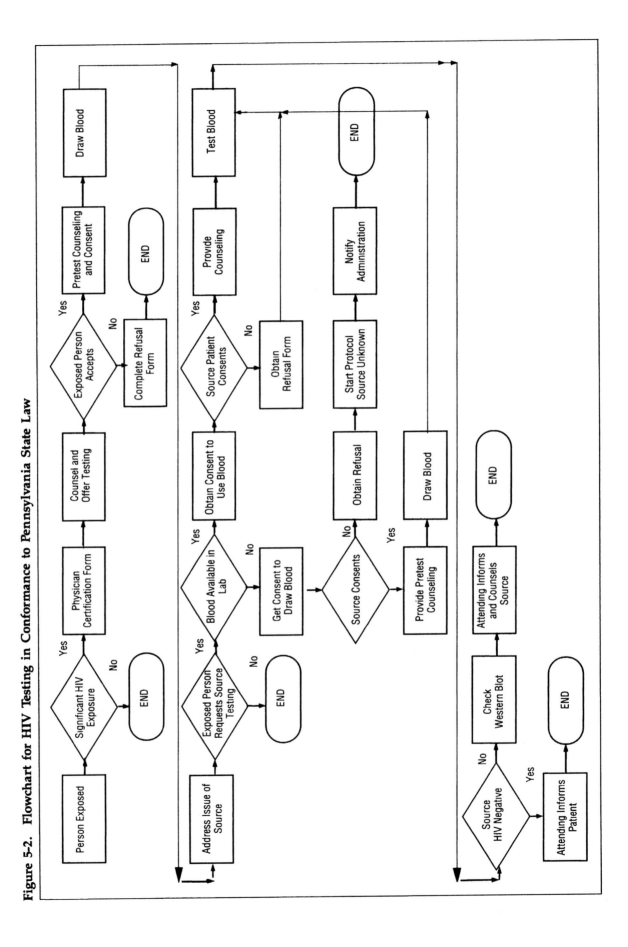

Figure 5-2. Flowchart for HIV Testing in Conformance to Pennsylvania State Law

levels may or may not be sufficient to meet customer expectations and state-of-the-art professional standards. If the process were improved, they could do better.

For example, department heads at one midwestern hospital were angry year after year because their administrators encouraged them to propose improvements and innovations but then did not respond to the proposals. The department heads had become demoralized and cynical about the possibility of making important changes happen. Their disaffection and cynicism upset the administrators, who then decided to improve their decision-making process in order to better satisfy their customers, in this case, their middle managers. The improvement centered on meeting the department managers' expectation of "getting an answer in no more than three weeks." The result is clearly demonstrated by comparing figures 5-3 and 5-4. Figure 5-3 is a flowchart of the "current reality" as reported by department heads, and figure 5-4 is a flowchart showing the revamped process. Because the administrative team could not possibly meet the three-week time frame with their "current" decision-making process, they had to change the process itself in order to make the time frame feasible.

□ Conclusion

Operational requirements are the requirements of each step in the process designed to produce the output or service that the customer wants. These requirements should be determined on the basis of your understanding of the expectations and standards you are trying to meet, rather than on the basis of "how we've always done things here." If your current process is not capable of consistent conformance to these requirements, you need to take steps to redesign it. Over time, through continuous process improvement, you will narrow the gap between performance and requirements and push the standards upward, with the result that both customer satisfaction and optimal clinical outcomes will be achieved.

Figure 5-3. Flowchart Showing Current Decision-Making Process

Department head submits fully researched, complete proposal to his or her administrator. → Administrator loses it in in-basket. → Department head asks, "What's happening?" → Administrator says, "We're reviewing it."

Administrator finds proposal in piles on desk. → Administrator sends proposal to peer for review. → Peer loses it in in-basket. → Department head asks boss, "Where is it?"

Boss asks peer, "Where is it?" → Peer finds it in piles on desk. → The administrator and peer set up a meeting. → At the meeting, they deal with a crisis instead of the proposal. - - →

etc.

Weeks, months pass!

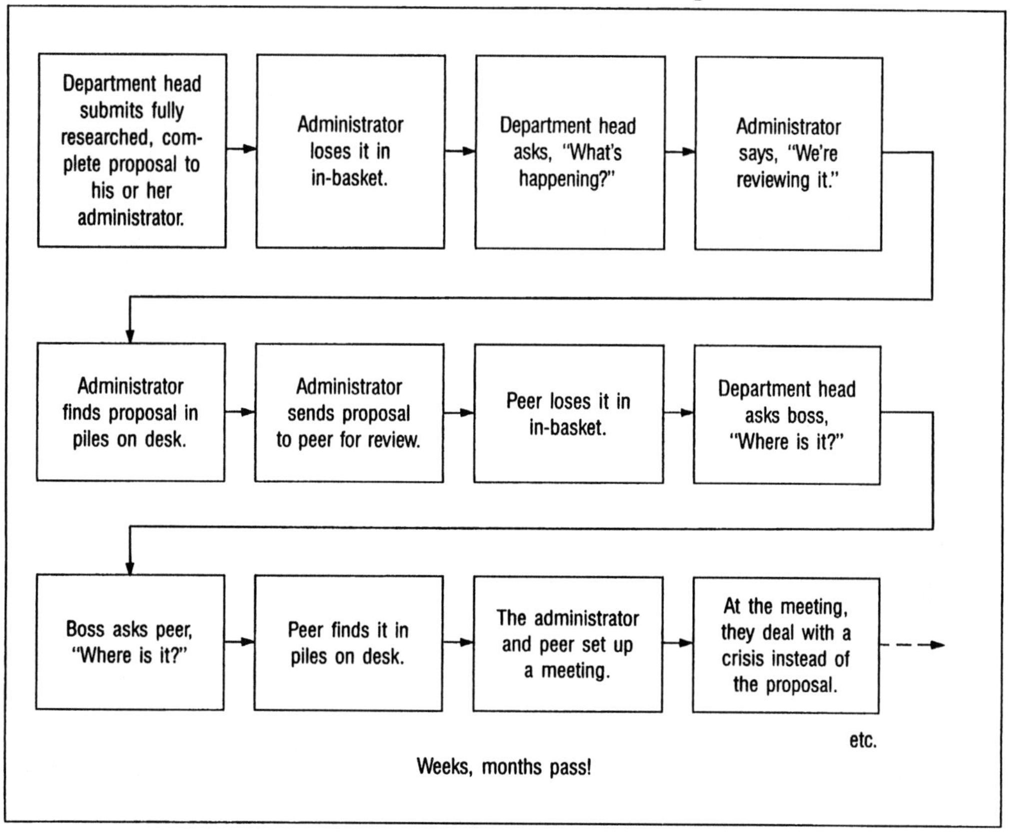

Figure 5-4. Flowchart Showing Improved Decision-Making Process

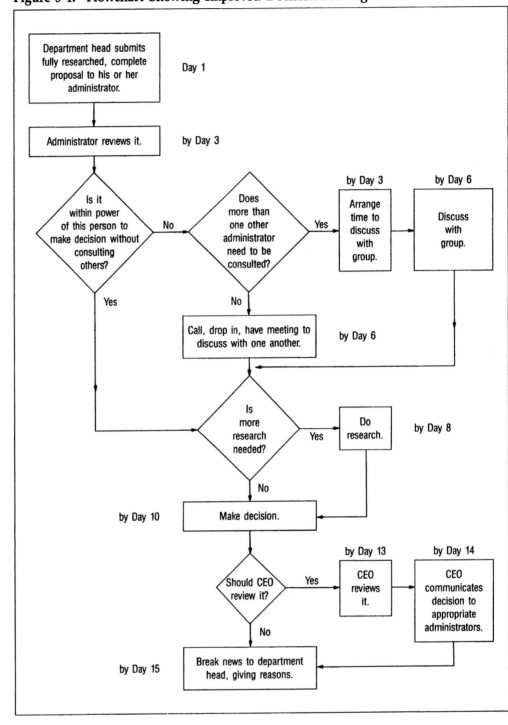

Chapter 6

Developing Measures to Monitor Performance

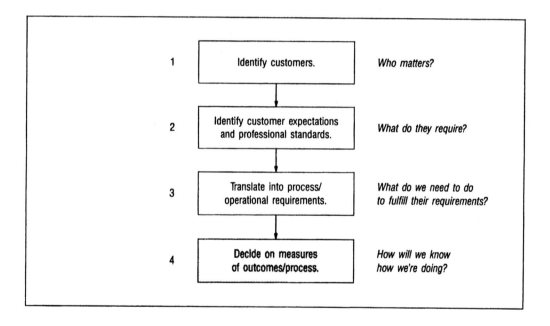

1	Identify customers.	Who matters?
2	Identify customer expectations and professional standards.	What do they require?
3	Translate into process/ operational requirements.	What do we need to do to fulfill their requirements?
4	Decide on measures of outcomes/process.	How will we know how we're doing?

Once you have begun to translate customer expectations and professional standards into process requirements, you need to establish an appropriate mix of measurement devices. These devices should enable you to monitor both the process and its results so that you can provide feedback to those with the power to make improvements. In short, you need to keep score as a matter of routine.

☐ The Importance of Feedback

In health care, feedback has historically been scarce. Our actions regarding what is best for our customers are based on our own views and those of professional groups, with few reliable means of discovering the customers' perceptions.

Most people become motivated to do better when they are provided with feedback about their current performance. Consider, for example, the difficulty of dieting without having a scale to measure progress. Most health care professionals who have been given legitimate feedback about their performance instinctively make efforts to improve it. And most work teams will value and devote energy to process improvement when, through measurement, they can see the results.

For example, at Kaiser Medical Centers in San Rafael and Santa Clara, California, leaders wanted to improve physician behavior toward health maintenance organization (HMO) members during office visits. Disappointed in the impact of educational programs designed to build the patient relations skills of their physicians, the leaders decided to implement a system of feedback that would enable them to give each physician information about his or her own patients' perceptions of the service they received. After visiting the physician, each HMO member completed a short "report card" rating the physician on several attributes. Each physician received a monthly summary of the data collected from his or her patients, along with a rank-ordered list (by number, not name) indicating where that physician's performance fell in relation to the performance of other physicians.

As a result of this very specific feedback, physicians improved their behavior significantly and immediately. They received data about their effect on their customers and, being dedicated health care professionals, they took steps to improve their behavior.

☐ Measurement Provides Control

To gather reliable, credible feedback, you need to measure, measure, and continue to measure. Measurements fulfill several essential purposes:

- They help us manage by facts, not opinions.
- They tell us how we're doing and motivate us to make improvements.
- They make accountability for continuous improvement possible and illuminate decision making by enabling us to set improvement priorities based on information rather than impulse or instinct.
- They settle differences of opinion among staff about performance.
- They provide information/evidence. You can't know whether you're winning or losing without a scorecard. Evidence of winning triggers pride and celebrations; evidence of problems sparks improvement initiatives.

Without measurement there is no control. By measuring operational performance, in particular, you can track variation and, when variation is beyond acceptable limits, attempt to reduce the sources of variation that are interfering with consistent quality performance.

☐ Step 4: Decide on Measures of Outcomes and Process

You do not have to be a measurement expert to develop measures of outcome and operational performance. Generally, it takes more common sense than technical training. Ask yourself the following questions:

- For satisfaction: What have we determined our customers' expectations to be? How can I get customers to tell us how well we are meeting their expectations?
- For direct measures of outcome: What evidence is available to tell us whether the output of our process met the customers' expectations? And what evidence is available to tell us whether the output of our process met our professional standards?

- For the performance of the process itself: How can we measure the key steps in the process that contribute to meeting expectations and standards so that we can control and improve them?

The following sections provide a framework for making specific decisions about what to measure and how to go about measuring it.

What to Measure

To achieve a complete picture of how your function is performing, you need to measure three things:

- Customer satisfaction
- Key attributes of quality deemed important to the customer and those defined by professional standards
- Performance of key elements in your processes, or critical control points

Organizationwide Measures

To create a context for this discussion and show how your department measurement plan connects with your organization's overall measurement plan, we should first look at the above three components as they are measured organizationwide. The pyramid in figure 6-1 describes a customer-oriented measurement system for your organization as a whole.

Overall Customer Satisfaction

At the top level, your organization might survey patients, family members, physicians, payers, and community members to determine their level of overall satisfaction with your organization (compared perhaps to your competitors). They might ask patients such questions as: "How likely would you be to choose our organization again if you needed health care services?" At this level, other organizational measures of overall quality might be the ratio of compliments to complaints, employee turnover, and dollars spent on rework.

Outcomes Related to Key Quality Attributes

At the midlevel, your organization would monitor each customer group's perceptions of the attributes of quality important to them—attributes that enter into overall satisfaction. So for patients, the organization might survey timeliness of service, courtesy of service, staff competence, and communication quality because patients tend to select these attributes as key to their satisfaction. For physicians, your organization might ask about

Figure 6-1. Measurement Pyramid for Your Organization

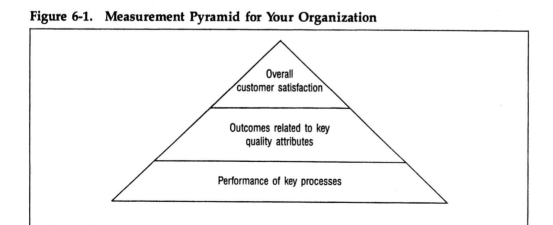

the turnaround time of lab, radiology, and other test results; the overall user-friendliness of the hospital; the quality of nursing care; and the responsiveness of the organization to physicians' needs because these tend to be the specific criteria physicians report as being important to their satisfaction.

Performance of Key Processes
At the lower, more specific, and more detailed level, the organization would measure the performance of key cross-functional processes that have a great impact on customers' perceptions of the attributes important to them. For example, because patients value timeliness of service, the organization might measure the timeliness of several key processes, such as admissions, discharge, nursing services, and so forth. Other measures at this level are shown in figure 6-2.

Department-Level Measures
At the department level, the measurement pyramid might look like the one shown in figure 6-3. For example, if you were the head of maintenance and engineering, one of your key customers would be the nursing services department. At the top level, you might survey the department monthly about its satisfaction with your department. At the middle level, you might ask for specific feedback about your performance on attributes

Figure 6-2. Some Measures of Performance at the Lower Level of the Organizationwide Pyramid

Valued Attribute	Measure/Indicator
Staff competence	Percentage of employees meeting performance standards
Quality of medical care	Percentage of nosocomial infections
	Percentage of unplanned readmissions to the emergency room, intensive care, or operating room within 48 hours
Timeliness	Percentage of customers waiting longer than departmental time standards for services, tests, information, calls
	Percentage of procedures not initiated within departmental time standards
Cost-effectiveness	Average cost per patient, adjusted for acuity

Figure 6-3. Measurement Pyramid for Your Department (for Each Key Internal and External Customer)

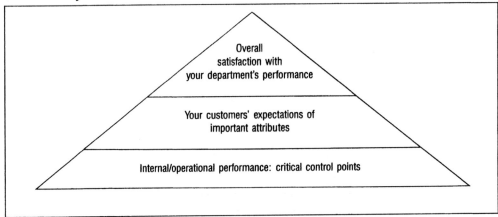

important to the nursing department, such as response time to regular requests for maintenance, response time to stat requests, and courtesy when nursing staff call with a question or complaint. Also, you would monitor the facts related to these important quality attributes. For example, you would log response time to completion for both routine and stat maintenance orders originating from nursing so that you could see exactly how long these processes take. Finally, at the lower, more detailed level, you would measure key steps in the process, or critical control points, for example, the time it took the receptionist to log in the order and convey it to a supervisor for delegation to the appropriate technician, the time it took the supervisor to assign the work, the time it took to secure the needed supplies, and the time it took to schedule and perform the work.

One nursing department identified pharmacy as a primary internal customer and interviewed that department about its expectations of nursing. Pharmacy was surveyed monthly to determine its overall satisfaction with nursing during the previous month. And, more specifically, pharmacy was asked to rate nursing on what it considered to be attributes of importance:

- Completeness of medication orders, without need to clarify
- Legibility of orders
- Appropriateness of stat orders
- Courtesy of nursing staff in telephone contacts

In order to monitor and improve the fulfillment of pharmacy's expectations, nursing set up internal measures such as:

- Quality checks on medication orders
- Criteria for stat orders and logging of conformance
- Protocols for telephone contacts and supervisory monitoring of conformance

Other nursing measures might include:

- Number of patients inadequately prepared for tests (for example, radiology, blood, and so on)
- Percentage of medications delivered to patients within departmental time standards
- Percentage of patients prepared for discharge within departmental time standards
- Percentage of patients able to accurately summarize discharge instructions within 48 hours of discharge
- Time from call light to nurse contact with patient

In billing, measures of customer expectations and professional standards might include:

- Percentage of bills accurate as audited
- Percentage of customer complaints
- Percentage of bills mailed within departmental time standards
- Percentage of customers satisfied with result of complaint call

In radiology, measures might include:

- Number of retakes needed
- Turnaround time of result to physician
- Number of complaints by referring physicians
- Percentage of patients seen within departmental time standards

- Patients' perceptions of quality of explanations, courtesy, and gentleness of technologists
- Quality of radiologist's reading as measured by a double-reading process

Other parameters to measure might be:

- Percentage of staff turnover (nursing)
- Percentage of documents accurate (medical records)
- Percentage of rework (tests, X rays)
- On-time delivery (storeroom, linen, dietary)
- Setup time (surgery)
- Rate of patient falls (nursing)
- Number or percentage of medication errors (pharmacy)
- Injury rate due to equipment problems (biomedical engineering)
- Percentage of reportable security incidents (security)
- Unplanned returns to operating room (surgery)
- Percentage of incomplete records (medical records)
- Percentage of rejected charges (third-party billing)
- Percentage of preregistered patients (admissions)
- Percentage of perfect documents (word processing)
- Percentage of on-time surgeries (operating room)
- Percentage of appropriate diagnoses (clinical department)
- Percentage of telephone pickups within three rings (any department)

How to Measure

There are many methods for measuring quality, both in fact and in perception, including surveys, logs, check sheets, time charts, histograms, and more. Most likely, you already have certain measures in place that you may want to reevaluate or augment. We suggest that you focus on one customer expectation and professional standard at a time and engage staff, peers, and/or experts in a creative discussion of how you might monitor performance related to those attributes in a way that is:

- Feasible or doable with your current staff
- Affordable
- Simple and straightforward
- Face valid (it measures what you want it to measure)
- Arithmetically sound
- Reliable (it remains consistent with repeated use)

To monitor customers' *perceptions*, surveys and face-to-face or telephone interviews work well. To monitor *facts* about timeliness or accuracy, rework, or other attributes of your work processes, simple check sheets and logs work well. Part III of this book provides a detailed discussion of these tools and their applications. You might also want to consult the professionals in your organization who are most experienced in measurement, including those in quality assurance, marketing, customer service, management engineering, risk management, and research.

Figure 6-4 is a summary of the discussions of a medical records department steering committee that had selected measures to track performance related to three expectations important to one of their customer groups—physicians. After considerable discussion about the cost of the various measures, the time involved in data collection and analysis, and the face validity of the resulting data, the group decided to monitor the first expectation (satisfaction with the timeliness of chart retrieval) with a question on a medical records report card or minisurvey distributed monthly to physicians. To measure fact as well as perception, the committee also decided to log actual chart retrieval time so that they could systematically control or improve it. To monitor the second expectation,

Figure 6-4. Measures to Track Performance Related to Three Physician Expectations of the Medical Records Department

---

**Medical Records Department
Performance Indicators Related to Physician Expectations**

Expectation 1. Timely retrieval of patient charts

1. Survey 20 physicians weekly. Use short, written survey question: "Overall, how quickly did medical records staff retrieve any charts you needed?"
2. Have physicians write "time of request" on chart request form. The clerk writes "time delivered" once chart is retrieved. Each week, the supervisor samples 100 forms and calculates number of charts retrieved within departmental standard of two minutes.
3. When asked for a chart, the clerk keys the time of the request into the computer. When the chart is delivered, the clerk keys in the time. Software produces daily and weekly summary report.

Expectation 2. Staff courtesy when the physician requests a chart

1. Include on the physician survey: "When you requested charts from our staff, how courteous were staff toward you (on scale from 1 to 6)?"
2. Log the number and nature of complaints about staff courtesy when physicians request charts.
3. Supervisors call three physicians a week to ask their perceptions of staff behavior when they request a chart.

Expectation 3. Convenience of opportunities provided for physician to sign attestation statements

1. Using a histogram, count the number of attestation statements signed within 24 hours, 24 to 48 hours, and so on.
2. Survey physicians on the convenience of signing attestation statements.

---

courtesy, the group logged complaints and included a question about staff courtesy on their so-called report card. To monitor the committee's own effectiveness in making the signing of attestation statements convenient for physicians (the third expectation), members tracked perception with this question on the report card: "How convenient was it for you to sign the chart?" Then, using a histogram to display the results, they tracked the outcome of convenience by recording how many attestation statements were signed within various time intervals.

To identify measures for your jurisdiction, start by generating several possible indicators for the variables you want to measure. Ask the following questions:

- Which attributes of satisfaction do we want to measure by soliciting customer perceptions? How can we measure these attributes?
- Which outcomes important to customers can we measure directly? How?
- Which professional standards can we measure directly? How?
- Which critical control points should we monitor to ensure that the process is working to produce these outcomes? How can we monitor these? (Then, do a trial run of these measures to make sure that you can make them feasible and practical within your department's everyday routines.)

☐ Involve Your Staff

Your staff is the key to measuring performance. First, invite staff members to share their perceptions of performance quality. This is important not only to supplement other measurements of performance, but also to engage the service providers—the people closest to your customers and your work processes—in the measurement and evaluation process. Second, engage staff in the collection of data.

When you engage staff in the measurement process, you engender a feeling of participation and interest in improving departmental and team performance. You constantly reinforce awareness about the attributes of quality important to your customers, directing staff attention to the pivotal elements in your processes that influence outcomes and customer satisfaction. You also counteract the resentment that some staff members feel when you install measurement and control devices that do not involve them and that make them feel that they are being watched and observed, not by peers but by authority figures or outsiders.

Invite Staff Perceptions

Focus groups or structured staff meetings are excellent methods for getting staff involved in decisions about what to measure and how to measure it. These methods not only help you increase employee participation in measurement, they also heighten staff awareness of what is important to their customers and how to detect evidence that their services are delivering it. Focus groups and structured staff meetings:

- Help you to identify in a rich, qualitative way the gaps that staff perceive between current service levels and those expected by your customers
- Show staff your respect for their experience and observations
- Refocus staff on attributes important to your customers

Figure 6-5 provides an example of a discussion guide for a periodic staff focus group. There is a caveat, however. Although staff focus groups can be very helpful, they should not replace quantitative methods. Because focus groups provide qualitative, not quantitative, information, you cannot reliably use them to show comparative performance over time in a trend chart, for example. Focus groups complement other methods, including surveys, logs, and trend charts.

Engage Staff in Data Collection

To minimize the work involved in data collection, your staff members need to become data collectors. This is easiest to accomplish for the monitoring of processes because with logs, check sheets, histograms, and other such devices, staff can typically collect data at the same time they are doing their jobs. For example, the radiology receptionist can record the times patients enter the department and the times they are finally led into exam rooms for their tests. A chart reviewer in medical records can complete a checklist of missing elements on patient charts. A tray delivery worker from dietary can ask patients how satisfied they were with the day's lunch.

Figure 6-5. Discussion Guide for a Periodic Staff Focus Group

Introduction: We met with our customers to identify their primary expectations of our department. Now we're trying to pinpoint how we're doing in relation to their expectations. Because you're close to the action, I know you can tell us a lot about the fit or gap between our customers' expectations and how we are currently doing.

Questions:
1. Our customers said _____ is important to them. How do you think we're doing on that?
2. How are we on course?
3. How are we off course?
4. What changes do you think we should make to better satisfy this customer expectation?

Proceed with similar questions related to additional customer expectations.

(To conduct staff focus groups, see the detailed instructions in chapter 10.)

Staff can also be helpful in collecting and tabulating information directly from customers. For example, the head of the radiology department at a particular hospital wanted her staff to become more attuned to customer needs. She created a system by which every staff member conducted a very brief interview (three questions, one per expectation) with three customers per week. Staff turned in their raw data and a clerk tabulated the data for everyone. Although the reliability of this technique may be questioned because of the number of interviewers, you can reduce variability by developing language protocols that everyone uses and by providing a forum for training and practice that helps staff members polish their approach.

However, the ultimate purpose of this kind of data collection, that is, to drive continuous improvement, should not be lost. By structuring staff–customer interactions in which the staff member is the nondefensive listener, the data-collection experience itself motivates staff members to take whatever steps they can to improve performance, either by improving their own performance or by suggesting improvements that will better satisfy their customers.

☐ Conclusion

In 1883, Lord Kelvin said, "When you can measure what you are speaking about, you know something about it; but when you cannot measure it, your knowledge is of a meager and unsatisfactory kind." By heeding this insight, you can build your department's performance on a solid foundation of both fact and perception. You will know how you are doing, and so will your staff. You will have a sense of direction for making improvements. And you will be able to monitor progress and see the benefits of your persistent efforts to make things better for your customers while meeting your professional standards.

Chapter 7

Using Data to Target Improvement Needs

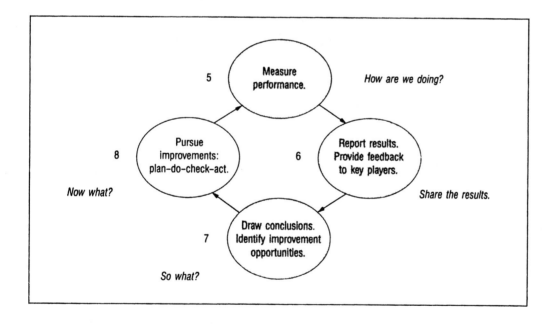

Once you have identified the measures for monitoring process and outcome, you can begin the ongoing, cyclical process of measuring, reporting, and using your findings to identify and pursue improvement opportunities. Without building this kind of cyclical process into everyday operations, you run the risk of using reactive, rather than proactive, problem solving. However, by methodically and routinely focusing on the cyclical process of continuous improvement:

- You can rationally select your improvement priorities by drawing on performance data, instead of responding to the most glaring crisis.
- Your attention will be on making enduring process improvements, not on putting a paint job on a machine that needs body work.

- You will feel more in control as a manager because you are *choosing* your improvement priorities rather than expending all your energy putting out fires.
- You and your staff will eventually recognize breakthroughs as you see the cumulative effect of many incremental process improvements.

☐ Step 5: Measure Performance

In order to measure performance, you need to design a regular schedule of measurement so that measurement becomes part of your routine and not a periodic headache or afterthought. How often you measure depends on your level in the organization and the purpose of your measurement devices. The closer you are to the customer, the more often you should measure so that you can make immediate course corrections in time to prevent problems from escalating. The pyramid shown in figure 7-1 offers some guidelines for measurement frequency, although you must ultimately determine your own schedule based on your resources, the difficulty of data collection, and how often you will realistically be able to review and act on the results.

Figures 7-2 and 7-3 (p. 66) present sample work sheets that may be useful in summarizing and making public your plan for tracking performance related to your customers' expectations and professional standards. In the Measurement Plan Work Sheet (see figure 7-2), you list in the left-hand column the indicators you plan to use to monitor outcomes and critical control points. Then, for each indicator, you show who is responsible for seeing that the measure is used regularly and appropriately, how often measurement should take place, who will actually collect the data, who will summarize them into a usable form, and which tools will be needed (for example, computer, checklists, survey questions, tally sheets, and so on) in order to implement this indicator as planned. Then, in the Measurement Schedule Work Sheet (see figure 7-3), you show your coordinated schedule for all measurement. At a glance, you and your staff will be able to see which measures are supposed to be used each week.

An example of a multipurpose tool that serves as a measurement calendar, shows thresholds for action, and displays results as they are collected is shown in the quality report used by St. Clair Hospital's Department of Medicine (see figure 7-4, p. 67). The department manager, director, or physician puts an X in those time frames when monitoring should occur. Once data are collected, the actual results replace the Xs. This format also lends itself well to computer spreadsheets and graphic trend charting of the data as they are collected over time.

☐ Step 6: Report Results and Provide Feedback

Data are meaningless unless they get into the hands of key players—the people with the power to act on the data. These key players include you, your staff, senior management, and any teams organized to pursue improvements.

Resistance to Information Sharing

Some managers collect valuable data but then hold the data close to their chests because they are afraid that disappointing performance will reflect badly on them. Or perhaps such managers feel more in control when they know more than others do about performance and outcomes. Or possibly they just do not remember to share the information.

The Fear of Sharing
If you are afraid to make performance data available to the appropriate individuals, there may be a force in your organization's culture that fosters fear. A guiding principle within Deming's 14 points is "drive out fear."[1] If you fear repercussions from data that show bad news, speak to your superior about it. Admit your concern and try to obtain a

commitment of support for your efforts at continuous improvement, including the sharing of data about performance with key people.

The Need to Control

If you hesitate to report results to your staff because you feel as though you're relinquishing control, consider the costs of withholding this information. How can your staff develop and continue to improve their performance when they are kept in the dark? When you withhold information, they most likely restrain their commitment, thinking, "If my boss thinks we're too dumb or too untrustworthy to understand this information and use it constructively, then let my boss make the improvements around here! Count me out."

Figure 7-1. Pyramid Showing Frequency of Measurement as Related to Organizational Level

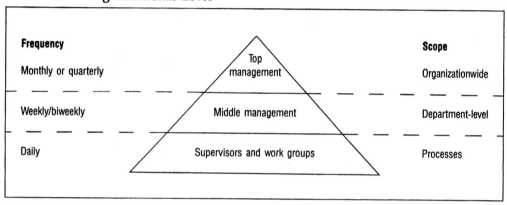

Figure 7-2. Measurement Plan Work Sheet

Measurement Plan for _____
Customer Group

Satisfaction indicators	Responsible manager/ supervisor	Data collected— how often?	Data collected— by whom?	Data summarized— by whom?	Tools needed	Notes
Process indicators						

Reprinted, with permission, from St. Clair Hospital, Pittsburgh, 1990.

Figure 7-3. Measurement Schedule Work Sheet

List the indicators and place a check mark in the weeks they are scheduled for implementation.

Indicators	Week																									
	1	2	3	4	5	6	7	8	9	10	11	12	13	14	15	16	17	18	19	20	21	22	23	24	25	26
1 Patient written survey																										
2 Patient focus group																										
3 Etc.																										
4																										
5																										
6																										
7																										
8																										
9																										
10																										
11																										
12																										

Figure 7-4. Example of a Quality Report Used by St. Clair Hospital

Year _____ 1990 _____
Department _____ Medicine _____

Activity	TFE	JAN	FEB	MAR	APR	MAY	JUNE	JULY	AUG	SEPT	OCT	NOV	DEC
Scope of care													
Referred occurrences	—	4	2	0	2	2	1	0	1	1	0	X	X
Referred mortality	—	1	0	0	1	0	0	0	0	0	0	X	X
Specific indicators													
A. Cardiac disease													
1. TPA effectiveness	70%			71%		91%		88%		X		X	
2. TPA appropriateness	95%			90%		100%		100%		X		X	
3. Art line indications	95%			100%		100%		99%					
4. Art line complications	1%			9%		4%		3%					
5. Swan-Ganz indications	95%			100%		100%		100%					
6. Swan-Ganz complications	1%			0%		0%		0%					

X = scheduled activity; TFE = threshold for evaluation; — = TFE not established

Reprinted, with permission, from Clara Jean Ersoz, M.D., St. Clair Hospital, Pittsburgh, 1990.

67

The Lack of Methodology

If you believe in sharing data with staff but do not have a reliable way to do it, you will benefit from using tools that make sharing information about performance a routine procedure. Such tools include written reports, posted trend charts, and regular meetings.

Whatever your resistance to information sharing, consider how you feel when your superiors withhold information and yet continue to expect responsible action, and sometimes even miracles, from you for the sake of the organization. Sharing information builds commitment and feedback drives improvement, instinctively and naturally. When feedback is negative, people want to make things better. When feedback is positive, people feel energized in their efforts to satisfy their customers.

Methods for Routine Information Sharing

To be effective, information sharing must become part of the routine, not an afterthought. Four methods of information sharing, or reporting, are presented here. Used individually or in combination, they can help keep your staff and other key players informed about their performance:

1. Regular written reports
2. Posted trend charts
3. Routine meetings
4. Periodic summaries

Regular Written Reports

Once you have identified performance indicators, you can create and use a report format to share results with your staff. The report may take the form of a trend chart, a control chart, a histogram, or some other display device. (A complete discussion of these tools can be found in part III of this book.) For example:

- A trend chart summarizes performance at regular intervals. It lets you see whether performance is improving, staying the same, or dipping.
- A control chart shows every instance of performance in relation to a mean level, helping you to see the variability from instance to instance.
- A histogram shows the number of times performance fell within various intervals (for example, the number of patients who waited between 0 and 10 minutes, 10 and 20 minutes, and so on).

These reports should be distributed weekly, biweekly, monthly, or quarterly, depending on your monitoring schedule. An effective report includes:

- The charts clearly labeled and user-friendly
- A short summary of conclusions (for example, "We managed to increase our response speed by 6 percent this month")
- The implications of the data (for example, "That means we should congratulate ourselves for a substantial improvement over last month's performance" or "Because this score is substantially below our expectations, I'll be convening a team of people to investigate the problem. I want a representative from each shift to participate. Please see me to suggest team members")

This report is routine because it is distributed regularly. People should be able to rely on receiving it. If you do not make it routine, it will always be a burden and a production—and therefore much less likely to happen. If you make it routine, you will figure out a way to build it into your department's regular cluster of activities.

Posted Trend Charts

Progress plotting is a powerful reinforcement device. Trend charts are especially powerful vehicles for communicating about performance levels. One department director decorated the wall outside his office with huge trend charts similar to the one shown in figure 7-5. Another department head used bar charts to show each month's actual performance compared to the department's goal, or target, and to the average performance for the three preceding months (see figure 7-6, p. 71).

Usually, at least one member of a work group enjoys making multicolor charts and will be happy to do the work involved. Also, user-friendly computer software is available to make bar and line graphs and charts (for example, Microsoft Excel™, Chartmaster™, Harvard Graphics™, Lotus™, DrawPerfect™, and a wide variety of statistical process control software).

Routine Meetings

Part of the time spent in staff meetings should focus on the collected data. By routinely devoting meeting time to performance feedback, you reinforce the value you place on quality and continuous improvement. You also build staff accountability and ownership in improving work processes.

Monthly meetings can be held expressly to review performance data; or a segment of every staff meeting can be devoted to examining recent reports, discussing their implications, and determining any actions to be taken. A possible meeting format might be the following:

- Ask people to guess how they think the department did on each indicator during the period in question. An occasional prize for the best guesser can build suspense and enhance interest.
- Show the results. Give people a chance to digest and discuss them. Answer questions as needed.
- Ask people to draw conclusions. Ask them how they interpret the results and what they see as the possible causes.
- Focus people on action that can be taken to improve the results (for example, assign certain problems to improvement teams, brainstorm possible experiments for improving performance, and so forth).
- Establish a target for the next time period (for example, "Let's see whether we can raise this by 2 percent if we institute the change we just designed").

Periodic Summaries

To see the big picture and present the improvements reflected in your data, periodic summaries of all your improvement efforts should be produced and distributed to staff. These summaries help people see a profile of performance across several indicators. The quarterly improvement summary shown in figure 7-7 (p. 71) is an example of such a report format. For example, if staff courtesy were an expectation, it would be entered in the column under "Expectations." The "problem" might be a curt telephone voice; a "cause" might be divided attention between callers and patients in the waiting area; an "action" could be securing telephone backup, and a "process lesson learned" might be that contingency plans need to be built into the process.

After summarizing the data and extracting meaning from them through effective reporting, you will be in a strong position to draw conclusions and institute course corrections that will improve performance. Also, determine whether people in other parts of the organization might benefit from the data you have collected and the changes you are making as a result. Share the wealth so that appropriate people in other departments can also be guided by the fruits of your labor.

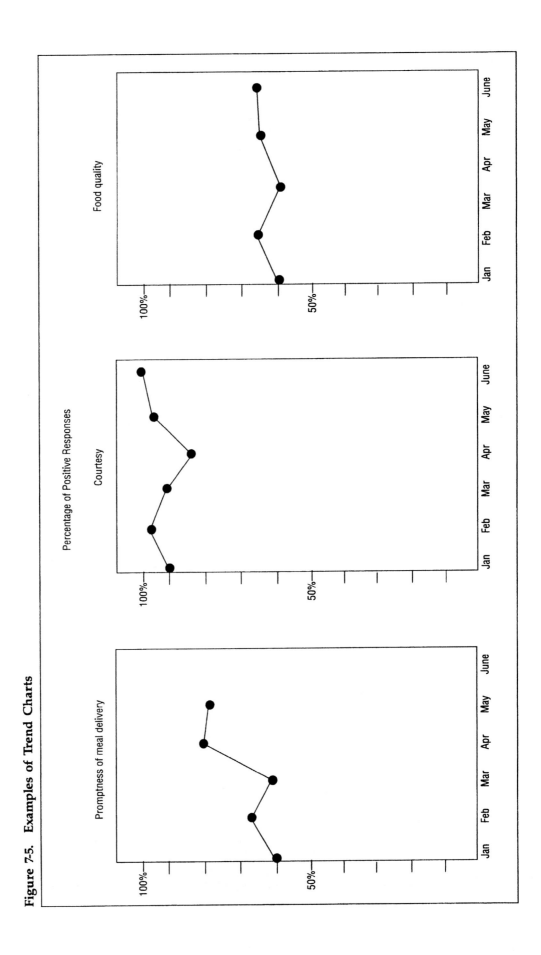

Figure 7-5. Examples of Trend Charts

Figure 7-6. Examples of Bar Charts Comparing Actual Performance with Target Performance and Previous Time Period

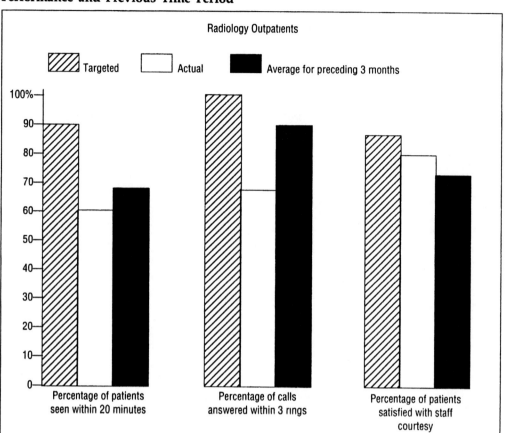

Figure 7-7. Sample Quarterly Improvement Summary

Expectations, requirements	Problems	Causes	Actions	Process lessons learned
1.	1.a 1.b	1.a 1.b 1.c	1.a 1.b	1.a 1.b
2.	2.a 2.b			
3.	3.a 3.b	3.a	3.a	3.a

☐ Step 7: Draw Conclusions and Identify Improvement Opportunities

Now you are ready to make sense of your results and figure out which problems or improvement opportunities merit corrective action or attention. Key questions at this stage include:

- What do we see happening regarding customer satisfaction? Are key customers more or less satisfied? What conclusions can we draw about the satisfaction levels of our customers?

- What do we see happening regarding our effectiveness in meeting our professional standards?
- How are we doing at critical control points in our process? Worse? Better? The same?
- Are there simple explanations or special causes of unusual results? If so, what do we need to do about them? If not, what processes do we need to improve in order to make enduring improvements?

After generating improvement opportunities, you can use voting, Pareto charts, and decision matrices to set priorities for improvement.

Voting

Voting among alternative improvement opportunities reflects a belief that all improvements are worthy and important and that staff will be eager to solve the problems they vote for or prefer. A concern, however, is that people might choose an easy or nonthreatening problem instead of the improvement opportunity most important to your overall effectiveness.

Pareto Charts

Pareto charts help you to distinguish between the *trivial many* focal points for improvement and the *vital few* by displaying them so that they are clearly arrayed in descending order of importance. By focusing your improvement efforts on the vital few, you use your time more efficiently. For example, if you administer a customer survey, you could decide to identify and seek to improve the worst result. The Pareto chart in figure 7-8 shows the results of a survey in declining order of importance. It shows that timeliness of service yields the highest percentage of dissatisfaction ratings (about 65 percent). Therefore, the group would be wise to devote its finite and precious time working to significantly reduce this.

Figure 7-8. Example of a Pareto Chart for Setting Improvement Priorities

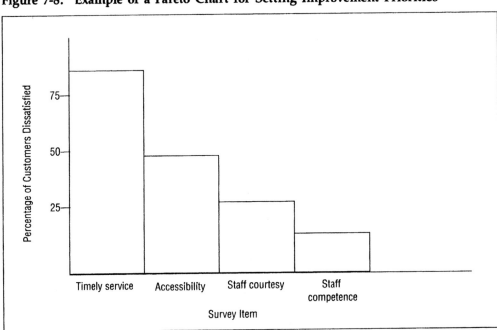

Decision Matrices

A decision matrix is particularly useful in selecting among alternative improvement opportunities. With a decision matrix, you first decide on criteria for narrowing down the number of improvement opportunities and then have group members rate the various alternatives according to these criteria. The criteria should reflect your particular realities, such as "must cost nothing," "can probably be accomplished without involving people in other departments," or "is a very high priority for the customer group involved."

For example, a radiology work team used a decision matrix to select a focus for problem solving (figure 7-9). The team members decided to rank order their alternatives according to three criteria: likely impact on the customer, likely impact on the staff, and likely ease of solution. They then totaled the numbers and picked the alternative with the lowest total, which was equivalent to the top-ranked alternative.

By *consciously* choosing among alternatives and using the tools of quality improvement, you will identify the improvement opportunities of greatest importance and benefit.

Figure 7-9. Example of a Decision Matrix for Selecting Improvement Opportunities

1 = highest, 3 = lowest				
Alternative improvement objectives	Impact on patient satisfaction	Impact on staff	Likely ease of solution	Total
Reduce patient scheduling errors	1	2	2	5
Speed up telephone response time	3	3	1	7
Find way to get pictures read faster	2	1	3	6

☐ Conclusion

With a manageable agenda of improvement opportunities now in hand, you can proceed to step 8 and pursue process improvements that will produce important gains in performance. Having followed the first seven steps of the customer-driven management process, you are now equipped to spend your valuable time homing in on specific high-priority problems because your viewpoint has been enlightened by meaningful information grounded in a solid understanding of your customers' expectations and the professional standards that must be met in order to fulfill these expectations.

Reference

1. Deming, W. E., *Out of the Crisis*. Cambridge, MA: Massachusetts Institute of Technology, Center for Advanced Engineering Study, 1986.

Chapter 8
Making Improvements

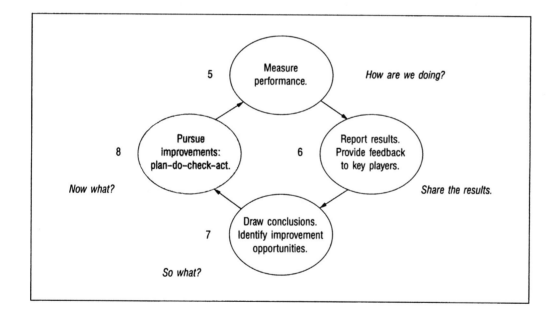

Pursuing and making improvements is the final step in the customer-driven management model. You have identified your customers, their expectations, and the relevant professional standards; and you have translated these expectations and standards into process requirements and decided on indicators for measurement. You then begin to implement your plans and decisions on a regular basis. You regularly measure your current performance, report the results to key players, and draw conclusions from the collected data that enable you and your team to identify the improvement opportunities that are priorities. The last step in this iterative process is to make concrete improvements, specifically, *process* improvements, in a rational and efficient manner. Focusing on a specific process needing attention, you now take steps to ensure that you are "doing the right things" in your efforts to achieve ever-higher customer satisfaction. This last step is where you actually pursue concrete, specific problems and opportunities for improvement.

☐ Step 8. Pursue Process Improvements

For years, health care organizations have focused extensively on performance improvement. For example, guest relations strategies have typically focused on helping staff improve their behavior toward their internal and external customers. Productivity strategies have focused on helping people get more work done faster. Although performance improvement is certainly important, without a powerful and complementary strategy to improve processes, there exists the risk of helping people do the "wrong things" better and faster. For that matter, all work at all levels needs to be seen as a process. The cartoon shown in figure 8-1 serves to explain (and demystify) what we mean by a process and how processes differ from performance and systems.

What Is a Process?

A process is a sequence of interrelated activities that convert inputs from suppliers into outputs for customers. Every process has suppliers, inputs, outputs, and customers. Inputs can include people, material, equipment, methods, and measurements. Consider a patient needing an X ray. Inputs into the process are the patient, the X-ray equipment, the film, the exam room, the staff members who provide the service, and the physician's order for the test. The suppliers of these inputs are the transporter who brings the patient to the lab for X ray, the vendors who sold the hospital the X-ray equipment and the film, the hospital that provided the physical space, and perhaps the personnel department that hired the staff who participate in the process.

Suppliers and inputs need to be identified when describing a process because quality problems might begin with them. If the equipment is defective, the process will break down; if the transporter has not delivered the patient on time, the process may be upset; if the film is defective, the process cannot be effective; if staff are untrained, errors may occur.

Some inputs are tools and some are raw materials that will be converted by these tools into outputs. In our example, the equipment (an input) is a tool that will convert the film (another input) into a picture of the patient's hip (an output). The process itself, then, either uses these inputs to help create the outputs needed or changes these inputs to produce outputs.

Every process has outputs and recipients of these outputs—the process's customers. Just as inputs comprise every thing and every person that influences the process, the outputs and customers include every thing and every person affected by it. The main outputs and customers in our example include a readable X ray image for the radiologist (the customer) to interpret; an entry into the patient's chart, which interprets the X ray in light of the patient's condition (for the patient's physician as customer); the patient, whose X ray has been taken and who is ready to return to his or her room; and the paperwork that triggers the X-ray charge to the patient's bill for the billing department (as customer). As you can see, some of the customers of the process are external customers (the physician and the patient) and others are internal customers (the billing department).

It is important to specify the outputs and customers in portraying a specific process because outputs are the goals of the process and help you to test whether the process is indeed producing the results the customer needs. By specifying who the customers are, you are aided in clarifying the outputs important to each.

To describe a process fully, then, you need to identify your suppliers and the inputs they provide and your customers and the outputs they expect, as shown in figure 8-2 (p. 80). By streamlining and strengthening the processes by which people do their work,

Figure 8-1. Cartoon Illustrating the Concept of Process

It all began when we looked at

PERFORMANCE

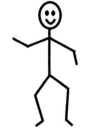

(Individual Actions)

The activities and behaviors that each individual does to serve customers at the highest levels of excellence.

Performance: "Actions designed to meet customer expectations."

But we soon learned that no individual's performance really stands alone. Each action is actually a "Performance Step" in a series of performance steps.

"a cog"

Each activity is a "cog" in a bigger picture . . . a picture that we began to call a . . .

PROCESS

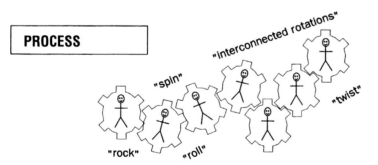

Actions connected to other actions . . . each step dependent on others. We can't just improve performance—we also *must* look at how to improve the *lineup* of actions and how the connections are working.

Process: "A series of interconnected and interdependent performance steps— designed to meet customer expectations."

(Continued on next page)

Figure 8-1. (Continued)

But again we knew that processes seldom if ever stand alone.

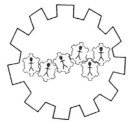

Each one is itself a "cog," part of an even bigger picture, connected to other process cogs in what we started to call a . . .

SYSTEM

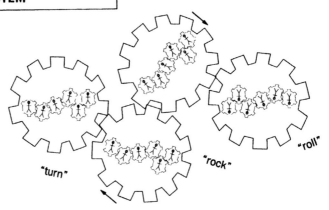

Where one process ends, another begins, each one serving customers who may even be other processes.

System: "A network of interconnected and interdependent processes— designed to meet customer expectations."

Figure 8-1. (Continued)

And *systems* themselves seldom if ever stand alone. They too are "cogs," interconnected parts of even bigger, more complex "macro" systems, systems that we call . . .

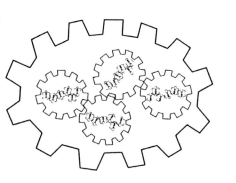

ORGANIZATIONS

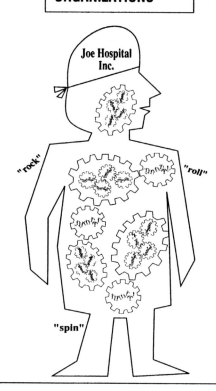

So hospitals are complex "systems of systems," interconnected and interdependent systems, processes, and performance all working to meet customer expectations. Quality performance, quality processes, quality systems in an "Organizational Culture of Quality."

Organization: "A system of systems. A complex collective *entity* of interconnected and interdependent systems—designed to meet customer expectations."

Reprinted, with permission, from the Einstein Consulting Group, Philadelphia, 1991.

Figure 8-2. Graphic Showing Process as a Sequence of Steps

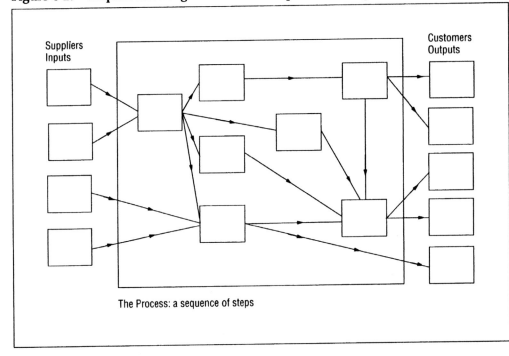

The Process: a sequence of steps

you will dramatically improve the quality of your results and reduce inconsistencies that are built into and produced by the process itself. For cross-functional or interdepartmental processes, this means a shift from a turf orientation to a process orientation that drives people to streamline and smooth out the interrelationships across departmental and functional lines. The graphic in figure 8-3 demonstrates the shift needed. On the left, solid lines represent the walls that so often exist between departments and cause breakdowns and barriers to quality performance and process. These turf lines make it difficult for outputs (results, people, paper, supplies, and the like) to flow unimpeded across lines. On the right, solid lines represent smooth, streamlined, tight processes that allow outputs to flow unimpeded across departmental boundaries.

In a quality organization, the processes integrate with other processes to constitute systems that allow patients, paper, supplies, requests, communication, and other outputs to flow smoothly across departmental and job lines and from process to process—all in the service of customers. Ultimately, you achieve a seamless system wherein multiple processes flow smoothly into one another.

Why Process Improvement?

As this book has repeatedly emphasized, the greatest payoffs result from a focus on process improvement. By improving processes, you improve the work or performance of many people and you expand the capability of your processes to produce high-quality results in less time, at lower cost, or with greater positive impact on your customers. When you clarify and improve a process, you always improve results.

The three primary goals of process improvement are:

- *Effectiveness.* Doing the right, appropriate things
- *Efficiency.* Doing these right, appropriate things right in minimum time and at minimum cost
- *Adaptability.* Resilience in responding to changing customer expectations and industry realities

Figure 8-3. Graphic Showing Shifts to Process Orientation

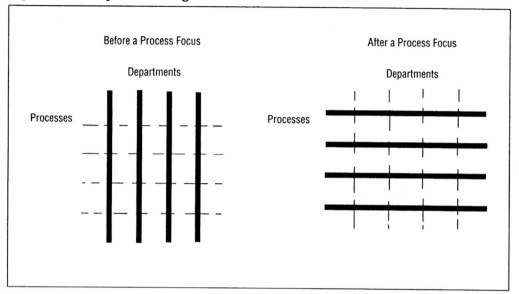

Stated another way, by improving processes you can:

- Improve the quality of care
- Increase customer satisfaction
- Minimize cost
- Minimize the time involved in delivering service
- Decrease staff frustration, empowering staff to be effective

This chapter presents a model for making specific process improvements. Some of the steps resemble those in the model for customer-driven management (identifying customers and outputs, setting up measures, and so forth). Here, however, these steps are applied to one specific process, not to overall departmental management. The model for process improvement works at the micro level; the model for customer-driven management works at the macro level.

The model for process improvement is an expansion of the plan, do, check, act (PDCA) system coined by Walter Shewhart[1] and promoted by W. Edwards Deming[2] (see figures 8-4 and 8-5 for Shewhart's model and an expanded version, respectively). First, you *plan* the improvement; then, you *do* it on a trial basis; next, you *check* or study it to determine the consequences or results; and finally, you *act* accordingly, if appropriate, building the improvement into everyday operations to standardize the process and hold the gains. Each of the four basic phases can be further broken down into substeps, as shown in figure 8-6 (p. 83).

☐ The PDCA Model for Process Improvement

Little is new about the PDCA model. It merely makes explicit and conscious the steps that many people intuitively and instinctively follow when making decisions and solving problems. Behavioral scientists often describe change as a three-step process:

1. Unfreezing, or thawing out established behavioral patterns
2. Changing, or moving to a new pattern
3. Refreezing, or maintaining the new pattern

Figure 8-4. Visual of the Shewhart PDCA Cycle

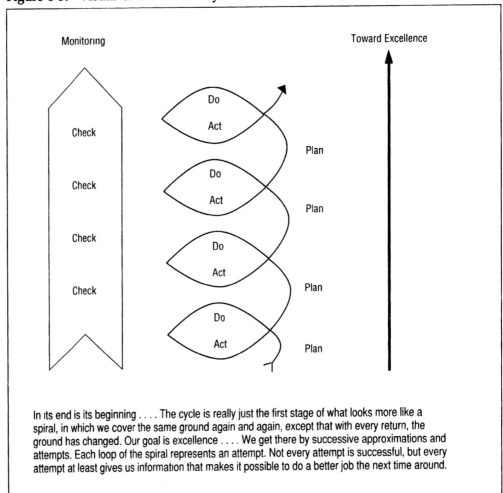

Figure 8-5. Visual of the PDCA Cycle as an Iterative Process

In its end is its beginning . . . . The cycle is really just the first stage of what looks more like a spiral, in which we cover the same ground again and again, except that with every return, the ground has changed. Our goal is excellence . . . . We get there by successive approximations and attempts. Each loop of the spiral represents an attempt. Not every attempt is successful, but every attempt at least gives us information that makes it possible to do a better job the next time around.

Figure 8-6. PDCA Model and Its 12 Substeps

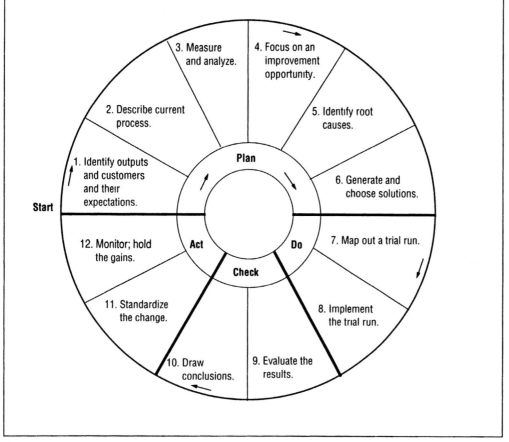

The PDCA model helps you to move yourself and your staff through these sometimes painful changes. To *unfreeze*, you acknowledge a problem or opportunity for improvement and investigate its ramifications and causes. You create a plan for improving things and take steps to gain a commitment to change on the part of staff and other powers that be. At the *changing* phase, you experiment, testing your proposed improvement in a trial run and closely monitoring its intended and unintended effects. Then, if you are convinced that the experiment worked and that the change is worth integrating into everyday operations, you move to the *refreezing* phase, in which you build in the changes and support people during what can be a disconcerting and unsettling process.

At each stage of the model, there are various tools you can use either alone, with a colleague, or within a team to clarify your thoughts and decisions. In chapters 10 and 11, versatile tools are described for use at the various steps (see figure 8-7). The following section examines each step of the PDCA model and the tools used in the process.

Plan Phase

In this phase, focusing on one specific improvement opportunity, you need to identify inputs, outputs, customers, and suppliers; crystallize customer expectations; describe your current process; home in on problematic aspects; test theories of causes; and identify solutions. Although there is a lot to do at this stage, which tends to be very time-consuming, thoroughness pays off.

Figure 8-7. The PDCA Model Including Implementation Tools

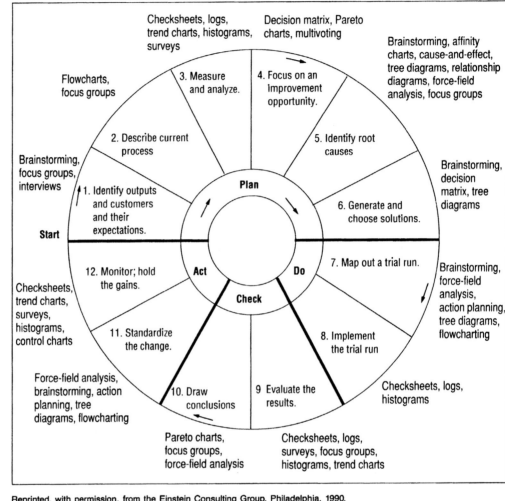

Step 1: Identify Outputs, Customers, and Customer Expectations

At this step, you ask questions similar to those you asked in the early steps of the customer-driven management process but with one important difference. In that process, you were asked to identify the primary customers of your department's overall functions on a macro level. However, at this stage, you are analyzing *one particular* process and should therefore specify the customers of that one process and the specifics about what they expect as outputs. This analysis is at a micro level. You are putting the customers and professional standards of one process under the microscope so that you can improve the process, with its specific recipients and their needs in full view.

The question here relates to the process itself and what it is intended to do. You need to ask, "What are we doing (the output)? For whom (the customer)? And what does the customer expect?" For example:

- What are we doing? Producing a test result. For whom? The physician. What does the physician expect? An accurate result quickly. Does *quickly* mean in minutes? In hours? In days?
- What are we doing? Completing paperwork. For whom? Medical records. What does medical records want? A record that is legible, complete, signed, and on time.
- What are we doing? Filling a prescription. For whom? Nursing first and ultimately the patient. What does nursing want? The right dose on time and clearly labeled.

- What are we doing? Providing linen. For whom? The patients. What do they expect? Clean linen regularly provided and within minutes if there's a mess.

To clarify outputs and customers, it helps to involve staff who have a hand in the process. To identify outputs, ask: "What are all of the outputs expected of this process?" You will generally arrive at a clear picture of your outputs, which you can fine-tune even further after flowcharting. To identify customers of the process, you ask: "Who receives these outputs?"

To determine customer expectations, you need to consult the customers of the process and determine their criteria for evaluating the outputs. Do they want no errors, a courteous interchange, legible handwriting, timely output, and so forth? The output of the process needs to fulfill these criteria in order for your customers to be satisfied. Methods to identify customer expectations were reviewed in chapter 4, which suggested that surveys and focus groups with customers are especially helpful. These tools are described in chapter 10.

Step 2: Describe the Current Process
After you have selected a process that needs improvement, it is important to achieve a shared understanding of how the process currently works. Who are the suppliers, and what are the inputs? What do we do now? What are the activities? In what order? What happens when things go wrong?

Nothing helps you to understand your current process better than flowcharting it. If you are working with a team, you can (and need to) use flowcharts to achieve a common understanding of the steps in the process so that you can identify specific improvement opportunities and develop theories about causes. You cannot improve a process if you cannot visualize how the process works in the first place.

In health care, many processes have evolved with no conscious design. When a team attempts to flowchart such a process, they find that there is no clarity about it; no one has an overview of how it is supposed to work. When this happens, if you persist in flowcharting the existing, albeit confusing and inefficient, process, you will quickly see possibilities for improvement, even possibilities for breakthroughs in performance. Deliberately designed processes are bound to work better than those that are invisible and out of control. By using the flowchart as a basis for creating a sensible discussion and data-collection plan, attention will become focused and endless discussion about causes will be eliminated.

Step 3: Measure and Analyze
Once you see your current process clearly, you can decide what data to collect and how to organize them so that you can better understand the performance and dynamics of the process. For example, if your problem is that patients leave the hospital feeling unclear about their condition and follow-up care, you might flowchart how communication with patients currently happens. The flowchart could help you to find out systematically what information is shared at each step, by whom, and with what degree of quality. Then you can check with patients *at each step* to find out how the problems or breakdowns occur.

The importance of flowcharting as a blueprint for beginning the measurement and analysis of your improvement opportunity cannot be overemphasized. Tools helpful at this stage for collecting and displaying data include check sheets, logs, surveys, trend charts, histograms, and Pareto charts. (See chapter 10 for an in-depth discussion of these tools.)

Step 4: Focus on an Improvement Opportunity
Within the specific process you are trying to improve, you can now home in on one improvement you want to make or one problem you want to solve. You can use multi-voting, decision matrices, and Pareto charts to help focus all the possibilities. This step

also resembles step 7 in the overall customer-driven management process explored earlier. The difference is that when you identified an improvement opportunity at step 7, you picked a *process* to improve. Here, you are working within the process to identify a *specific element* of the process to improve. For example, if you selected chart completion as a process that needs improvement, you might then focus your improvement efforts on the particular step in the process at which information from labs is entered on the chart.

Focusing on a specific step in the process you have identified for improvement is essential to your improvement effort. Many teams waste vast amounts of time because team members work at cross-purposes on different understandings of the problem. One clear, specific statement of the problem must be developed.

A good problem statement does a number of things. First, it states the effect that is unsatisfying, rather than theorizing about causes or implied solutions. It says what's wrong, avoiding such language as *lack of, due to,* and *we should.* It is simply a statement of the problem. Examples of some statements with implied solutions include:

- How to increase staff so patients do not have to wait so long in radiology
- How to double-check that medications are delivered to the right patient

Examples of some clear problem statements are the following:

- How to reduce patient waiting time in radiology
- How to reduce the number of medications delivered to the wrong patient

Second, a good problem statement:

- Focuses on the gap between current and desired reality
- Is measurable; states when and how much
- Is specific and tangible; uses concrete words, not vague concepts that mean different things to different people (such as *morale, communication, trust, attitudes*)
- Pinpoints the pain; emphasizes how customers, employees, and/or the organization are affected by the problem (for example, dissatisfaction levels, complaints generated, money wasted, and so forth)

To arrive at a good problem statement, it helps to generate many possible alternatives and then consciously choose *one* that is agreeable to everyone. A work sheet similar to the one shown in figure 8-8 could be used in the process. Team members compare notes about the symptoms of the problem and then generate alternative statements of the problem. They then discuss the alternatives and decide which problem statement they want to address so that everyone has the same focus. This process is helpful because many problems are multidimensional. For example, consider a problem first identified as a "morale problem." Trying to generate solutions without first establishing a clear focus would lead the team members in many different directions. However, answering questions such as the following on the work sheet would enable everyone to focus on the same problem:

- What are the symptoms of this morale problem?
  - We're losing talented staff.
  - People are grouchy and constantly complain.
  - We're hearing more complaints from patients than usual.
  - Unhappy staff people are dragging down their co-workers.
- Statements of the problem: The problem as I see it is . . .
  - How to increase retention of good people
  - How to improve the quality of our work life so that people aren't feeling so negative

Figure 8-8. Work Sheet for Pinpointing a Problem

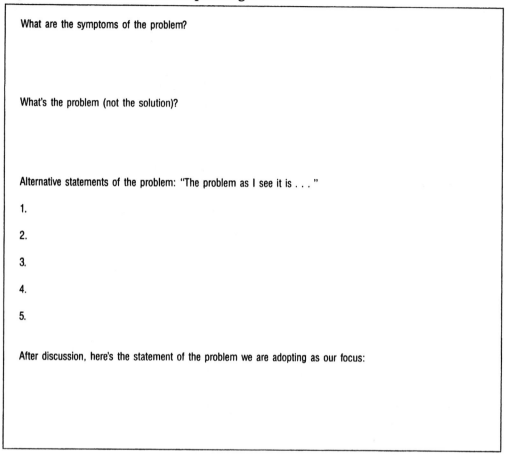

What are the symptoms of the problem?

What's the problem (not the solution)?

Alternative statements of the problem: "The problem as I see it is . . . "

1.

2.

3.

4.

5.

After discussion, here's the statement of the problem we are adopting as our focus:

—How to reduce the number of complaints from patients about our people
—How to increase the satisfaction level of our staff

As you can see, investigation of the problem and identification of solutions can be very different. In this case, it is clear that if the team skipped the step of selecting *one* problem statement, each member might be working with a different understanding of the problem, which would result in misunderstanding and confusion.

Typically, clear identification of a problem is an iterative process; it happens in successive approximations. At first, you might say, "The problem is, we frustrate our patients by keeping them in the dark about their medical condition." Then, after investigating the patients' information needs and the current process for meeting those needs, you determine that at the time of discharge, only 42 percent of your inpatients understand their condition and what they need to do to care for themselves at home. The problem may then be defined as "how to increase the percentage of patients who, at the time of discharge, understand their condition and home care instructions."

Step 5: Identify Root Causes
Once you've charted and analyzed your process and defined the specific problem, you need to generate and test theories about its causes. Most problems have more than one cause, but some causes have a more powerful impact on the problem than others. These are the root causes. Treating a root cause can reduce your problem significantly, whereas treating an "apparent" cause may do no more than relieve symptoms that eventually recur or reappear in some other form.

For example, patients may be frustrated by long waits in radiology. You cannot really resolve this problem unless you know why they are waiting so long. Are some staff out sick? Is the equipment down? Is the appointment scheduling system ineffective? Are patient charts not found until the patient arrives? Or some combination thereof? Any one of these facts might be a root cause of the long delays. Once you identify the root cause, you can design an enduring process improvement.

Three steps are helpful in identifying root causes:

1. Generate theories of causes.
2. Test these theories by gathering more data.
3. Pinpoint the cause(s) having the greatest impact on the problem.

For example, let's say patients and their family members think that the discharge instructions are confusing and incomplete. Using a cause-and-effect diagram and brainstorming, a work group or a team can identify the possible causes of this complaint. Causes may include:

- Pamphlets relevant to specific discharge conditions are not being consistently distributed to patients and their families.
- Patients and their family members who read the pamphlets do not find the information helpful.
- Patients only trust their physician to impart detailed home care instructions; yet, many physicians rely on the nurses to do this.
- Some patients and family members feel clear about discharge instructions at the time of discharge, but by the time they get home, they forget them.

These are theories about causes. Once you have generated theories, you usually need to gather more data to test them. In the preceding example, you might briefly interview patients just before discharge to determine how well they understand the discharge instructions and then later telephone them at home to see whether they have retained their understanding. That would test your theory that patients and their families feel clear about discharge instructions at the time of discharge but forget them by the time they get home. And to test your theories about the distribution and value of the pamphlets related to specific discharge conditions, you could follow up with a sample of patients to find out whether they received the appropriate pamphlet. The second phase of this follow-up would be to determine whether they read it. You could also ask them to read the pamphlet and evaluate the helpfulness of the information.

You can usually test your theories by simply asking, "How can we find out whether this is the cause of our problem?" Interviews with customers, observations of steps in a process, and discussions with other staff involved in the process can be helpful methods of testing your theories about causes.

You can then focus in on the one or two causes that exert the greatest impact on your desired results. This may be determined by listening to the people directly involved or examining the results of testing your theories and asking, "What does this say to us?" In the previous example, if patients read and understood the discharge pamphlet but disregarded what it said because "I do what my doctor tells me," the pamphlet is not the cause with the greatest impact. You would need to either help the physician give the pamphlet credibility in the patients' eyes or find a way to ensure that the physician can clarify discharge instructions personally, even though the pamphlet already summarizes them to the doctor's liking.

In some instances, you might select the cause with greatest impact by using a quantitative method, such as a Pareto chart. For example, if you were investigating the root cause of long delays, you could measure the time involved in each step of the process and determine the step or steps at which the longest delays occur.

Many simple tools are available to help you pursue all three steps in this cause identification process. To generate theories about causes, brainstorming, cause-and-effect diagrams, force-field analysis, the why–why form of a tree diagram, and affinity charts are especially helpful. Test your theories by collecting data through check sheets, logs, surveys, focus groups, interviews, and histograms. Then, use Pareto charts and relationship diagrams to select the root causes from among the several possible causes. (See chapters 10 and 11 for an in-depth discussion of these tools.)

Step 6: Generate and Choose Solutions

It is now time to think of solutions, preferably an array of possibilities. If you select one solution before you've generated alternatives, you often settle prematurely for the obvious and familiar in lieu of the powerful or creative. When working with a group, you need to set a tone that encourages creativity and wild-eyed possibilities and bans phrases and gestures that stifle the flow of ideas. As you may know, the idea of the steamboat was first ridiculed as Fulton's Folly; the atom was "irreducible," that is, until 1945; and in 1886, an eminent British surgeon declared that "surgery of the heart has reached the limits set by Nature—no new method and no new discovery can overcome the natural difficulties that attend a wound of the heart." In other words, there are innumerable possibilities that can be tapped if you create an atmosphere that encourages creative and uninhibited thinking and speculation about how things can be done better.

Helpful tools at this point include focus groups with customers and suppliers, discussions with the staff involved, affinity charts, and brainstorming. Then, focus groups, interviews with staff, and decision matrices help in selecting the most promising solutions from among the many.

Do Phase

At this phase, you plan and enact your pilot. To begin with, you need an "experimenter" mind-set. As yet, you do not have a solution; rather, you have a *proposed* solution, a well-researched hunch that now needs to be tested.

Step 7: Map Out a Trial Run

What may appear to be an exciting and brilliant solution may turn out to be off the mark. Therefore, you must take the pains necessary to execute it effectively and evaluate its worth. You need to secure whatever financial, technical, and human resources necessary for a trial run, and you need to involve the right people in accepting the idea and doing their part to implement it. That is why you must have a *plan of action* that includes implementation steps that indicate who is responsible at each step and by when, how implementation will be monitored, and how and when results will be verified. Such a plan is best developed by the people responsible for making the solution work so that their imprint is on the final outcome. Figure 8-9 shows a plan for revising (or improving) discharge planning instructions.

Step 8: Implement the Trial Run

Even after you have devised a great implementation plan, your work is not over. Often, people conclude that an experiment did not work when, in fact, it was never implemented as planned. Because you are introducing change and because old habits (processes) are difficult to change, you need to build monitoring and controls around your implementation process so that you *know* that what is supposed to be happening is actually happening. You cannot say the pilot failed if it was not thoroughly tested. Thus, when you implement the trial run, be sure to meet periodically with key players and observe and chart the process to ensure that implementation is conforming to plan.

Figure 8-9. Plan for Improving Discharge Instructions*

	Start	Finish	Who?
1. Collect current written materials	Week 1	Week 2	Pat
2. Convene physicians/nurses to review quality of old discharge instructions	Week 2	Week 2	Martha
3. Review with customers Pinpoint problems	Week 2	Week 2	Jack
4. Revise content	Week 3	Week 3	Pat/Jack
5. Show to customers; "pilot" draft; obtain feedback	Week 6	Week 8	Martha
6. Revise	Week 9	Week 10	Pat/Jack
7. Physician/nurse approval	Week 10	Week 11	Martha
8. Typeset/print	Week 12	Week 16	Kevin
9. Replace old with new discharge instructions	Week 17	Week 17	Cindy
10. Promote; send new instructions to nurses, physicians	Week 17	Week 18	Kevin/Jan

*The plan was to fix written brochures and checklists that describe discharge instructions for key categories of patients.

Check Phase

Once your experiment is in place, you need to monitor performance to evaluate results and determine the extent to which the changes are indeed making things better.

Step 9: Evaluate Results
Consult your process and outcome indicators to verify the effectiveness of your experiment. Control charts, trend charts, checklists, logs, check sheets, and simple observations are useful for this purpose. To understand the effects on internal and external customers' perceptions, surveys, focus groups, and interviews are especially useful. (Chapter 10 describes ways to use these tools purposefully during this phase.)

Step 10: Draw Conclusions
With evaluation results in hand, you're ready to make one of three decisions:

- The results look promising, but we have to fine-tune the changes.
- Our pilot failed; we need to go back to the drawing board and generate other possible solutions.
- It worked. Now it's time for us to make it routine!

Questions that help are:

- Did your change indeed produce improved performance?
- What are the costs and benefits of the improvement?
- Does it make sense to alter the everyday process to incorporate the changes made—to hold the gains?
- If so, what needs to be done to change the process? What modifications need to be standardized and *how* can people, materials, equipment, and schedules be equipped to make the transition?

Act Phase

At this stage, you do what is needed to integrate positive changes into everyday work processes so that your gains persist over the long haul (or until you make further improvements).

Step 11: Standardize the Change
Tasks at this stage include:

- Draw a revised flowchart and clearly show the revamped process as it should work from now on.
- Consider other areas in which the solution might beneficially be applied. Consult the people involved and determine the scope of the standardization process.
- Modify standards, procedures, policies, and performance expectations to reflect the changed process.
- Communicate the changes to the employees, customers, and suppliers involved.
- Train as needed.
- Develop a clear plan for supporting people throughout the change process; provide a supportive environment, create clear channels for reviewing snags and frustrations, and acknowledge and recognize changed behavior early on.
- Document the project, circulating its evolution or story (perhaps using a storyboard) to senior management, other department managers, the people who worked on the solution, other team leaders or facilitators who can learn from your experience, and the frontline people who will actually *do* the changed process in the future.

Caution: People often lose steam during this phase of the process and feel as though their job is done. As a result, they may not be as methodical or persistent in standardizing their changes as they need to be. It is true that the suspenseful, exciting phases of the detective work and problem solving are, for the moment, done. However, if you don't keep a tight rein on the process of internalizing your changes into everyday work, the gains will be lost. Your situation will regress to its former level despite the hours, days, and sometimes months spent correcting it.

At this stage, you need to plan, document, communicate, train, and monitor. Helpful tools include:

- Brainstorming sessions to discuss the steps involved in standardizing the process
- Flowcharts of the new process that can be used to orient and train staff to follow the process
- Clear, written instructions for specific steps in the process
- A troubleshooter's guide explaining what problems might be anticipated and how staff might handle them
- Training guides and opportunities followed by one-on-one coaching
- Implementation planning tools (see chapter 11)

Step 12: Monitor to Hold the Gains
To ensure that the changes stick, you need to continue a regular schedule of measurement and process control. Scatter diagrams, checklists, and run charts can help you monitor performance regularly at critical control points and comparatively over time.

For example, in one hospital the admissions department worked with housekeeping, nursing, and transport services to reduce admissions waiting time. After process improvements have been implemented to make it possible for patients to complete the admissions process, receive a room assignment, and be taken to a clean room by a transporter in a timely fashion, the process is monitored as follows: the admissions representative logs patient arrival time into admissions and the time it takes to escort the patient to his or her room. The representative calculates the "length of wait" and enters a data point for each patient on a run chart similar to the one shown in figure 8-10. To enable the patient to complete the admissions process and receive a room assignment, the admissions representative might use a checklist of steps to ensure that all tasks have been completed and the patient has been appropriately prepared for his or her arrival in a unit. Such a checklist might include the following steps:

Figure 8-10. Run Chart Showing Admissions Waiting Time

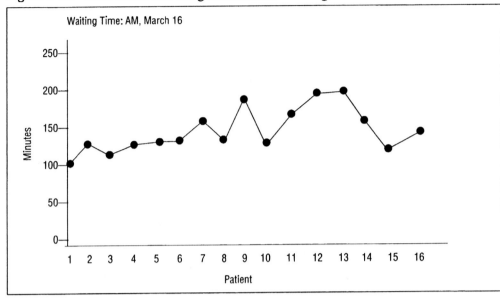

- Patient welcomed by representative and process explained
- Patient given "Welcome" packet
- Bed board notified to identify room assignment
- Room readied
- Registration process completed
- Patient received identifying wristband
- Transporter ordered
- Nursing alerted to patient's arrival
- Television clerk alerted to visit patient
- Switchboard notified of room assignment and phone number
- Physician notified of room assignment and other key information

Without such tools, hard-won changes often disappear because old habits die hard.

☐ The Model as a Guide

You may be thinking: "So many steps! So much to do! So complex!" Although we propose the preceding as a rational and sequential process, it is meant only as a blueprint or guide and not as a model to be followed lockstep. Our intention is not to make the improvement process tedious, nor is it to "program" you. As you proceed through the steps involved, you may find that you can skip certain steps because you already know the answers they will yield. However, be sure your answers are based on fact and not on opinion.

In proposing this model we had two options. One was to simplify and limit the number of steps to prevent your feeling overwhelmed by them. However, in considering that option, we found that a simple, short process excluded steps that were important in attacking *certain* problems. Excluding these steps would cause you to veer off course and waste time.

Therefore, we chose to present the option that involves more steps because it provides a more thorough, comprehensive process. Its advantages are clear. The steps are there if you need them so that you have the option of engaging in a particular step or skipping it. Before each step, ask the question, "Do we already know the answer that would result from this step?" If the answer is yes, move on; if the answer is no, do the step.

Simple and Obvious May Not Be Easy

Even after streamlining the process to fit the specific improvement you are pursuing, you might reach a solution that makes you think: "This is so simple. Can you believe we went through all that just to come up with this obvious solution!" But ask yourself, "If the change was so obvious, why wasn't it made before?" To unfreeze people from traditions and habits, it helps to go through steps that make them look at processes from a new perspective and commit to testing theories and making concrete improvements. It will sometimes take many meetings, tedious research, and precious time to come up with a seemingly obvious improvement, but the effort will help you to focus your attention and build confidence in the process change.

PDCA Thinking: A "Natural" for Health Care

For physicians, the PDCA approach to problem solving comes easily because it parallels the way they learn to approach the diagnosis and treatment of patients' illnesses. The chart shown in figure 8-11 reflects these parallels. This similarity in approach explains

Figure 8-11. The PDCA Cycle: A Natural Paradigm for Physicians

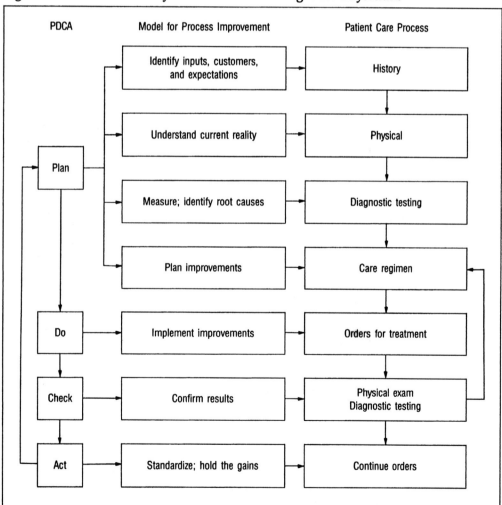

Reprinted, with permission, from Clara Jean Ersoz, M.D., St. Clair Hospital, Pittsburgh, 1990.

why many physicians find PDCA problem solving both comfortable and productive. In fact, many physicians become excellent improvement team facilitators because of their experience with the PDCA approach. PDCA thinking can also be seen in both the nursing process (see figure 8-12) and the Joint Commission's 10-Step Model for ensuring and improving quality throughout the organization (see figure 8-13).

☐ Conclusion

By making the implicit explicit and the unconscious conscious, you can gain control over your approach and *decide* what you need to do to pursue an improvement opportunity constructively. Just as a flowchart creates new possibilities for controlling and improving work processes, our model for process improvement, which is itself a flowchart, creates new possibilities for controlling and improving your effectiveness at process improvement.

As mentioned previously, it is not our intention that you should tediously follow every substep in this model in every case. However, we do want to point out that every step in the model serves an important purpose and may be useful in avoiding false starts, dead ends, and band-aid solutions as you pursue process problems. The chart shown in figure 8-14 (p. 96) summarizes the tools that are helpful at each step.

Figure 8-12. The PDCA Cycle: A Natural Paradigm for Nurses

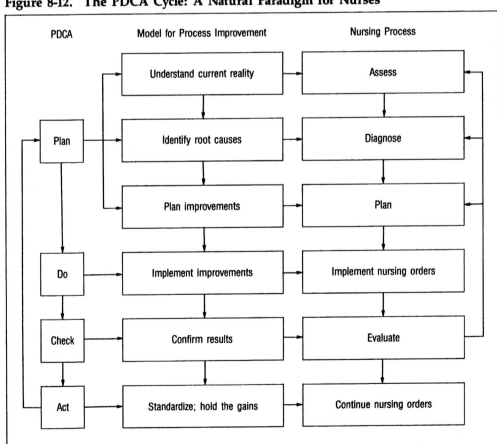

Figure 8-13. The PDCA Cycle and the Joint Commission's 10-Step Model

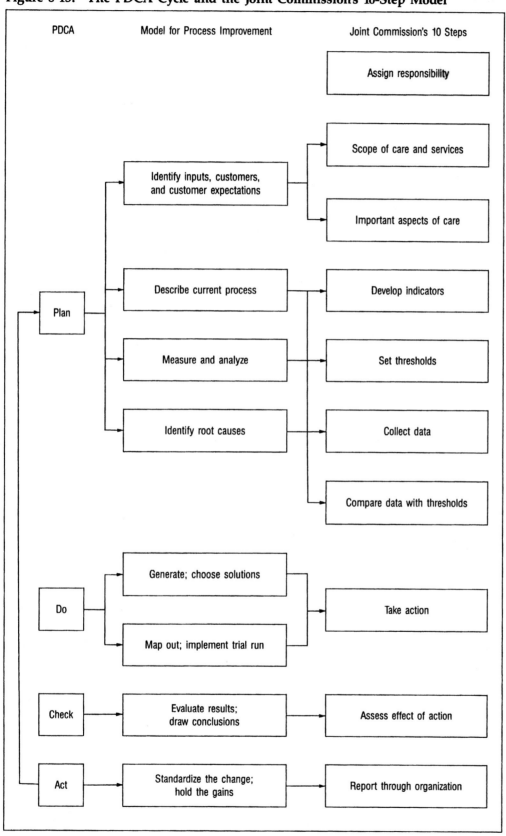

Reprinted, with permission, from Clara Jean Ersoz, M.D., St. Clair Hospital, Pittsburgh, 1990.

Figure 8-14. Guide to Use of Tools

	Identify outputs, customers' expectations	Describe current process	Measure and analyze	Focus on an improvement opportunity	Identify root causes	Generate and choose solutions	Map out a trial run	Implement a trial run	Evaluate the results	Draw conclusions	Standardize the change	Monitor; hold the gains
Focus groups	●	●		×		●	○		●	●	○	○
Surveys			●		○	○			●			●
Interviews	●	●		×	○	○	○		○	○	○	×
Check sheets			●					●	○			●
Logs			●					●	○			○
Histograms			●		○			×	○			×
Pareto charts				●	●					●		
Trend charts			●					●	●			●
Flowcharts				●	●	○	●				●	
Control charts			●					●	●			●
Brainstorming				●	●	●	○				●	
Affinity charts					○	×	○				○	
Relationship diagrams					●	○	○					
Cause-and-effect diagrams					●							
Force-field analyses					●		●		○		●	
Multivoting					×							
Decision matrices				○		●			○			
Action planning							●				●	
Tree diagrams			○		○	●	●				●	

● = Often used
○ = Used less often
× = Used rarely

References

1. Shewhart, W. *Economic Control of Quality of Manufactured Product*. New York City: Van Nostrand, 1931.

2. Deming, W. E. *Out of the Crisis*. Cambridge, MA: Massachusetts Institute of Technology, Center for Advanced Engineering Study, 1986.

3. Florida Power and Light. *QUALTEC Manual*. Palm Beach Gardens, FL: Florida Power and Light, 1989, p. 23.

Part III

The Manager's Tool Kit

Chapter 9

Introduction to the Tools of the Trade

T he old adage that "if you only have a hammer, you think every problem is a nail" attests to the fact that limited tools for quality control and problem solving mean limited effectiveness. We have learned from Deming and Juran devotees, as well as from Japanese and American businesses that have embraced the tools of continuous improvement, that managers can greatly enhance their effectiveness and save precious time by embracing a rich repertoire of analytical and creative tools data they can then use to tackle improvement opportunities.

☐ Tools of Continuous Quality Improvement

The tools of continuous improvement enable individuals and teams to achieve the following:

- Recreate complicated processes in picture form so that they can be surveyed and examined conveniently.
- Short-circuit what otherwise would be lengthy discussions in which only words would be used to manipulate multiple ideas. Graphics help people to manipulate many ideas much more rapidly than they could using words alone.
- Involve everyone quickly.
- Speed up consensus building and decision making.
- Improve the clarity and quality of results.

Resources on the tools of continuous improvement abound. In *Kaizen: The Key to Japan's Competitive Success,* [1] Masaaki Imai describes the seven quality control tools especially useful in identifying key causes, understanding processes, and measuring and tracking performance over time. Figure 9-1 is a visual presentation of these tools as shown in *Hoshin Planning: The Developmental Approach,* published by Goal/QPC. [2] In the 1970s, Yoshinobi Nayatani devised seven tools for management and planning under the auspices of the Japanese Society for Quality Control. These tools, also shown in *Hoshin Planning,* [3] extended the power and versatility of the more limited seven quality control tools. They are illustrated in figure 9-2 (p. 101). A wide variety of additional tools from different sources have also proved useful.

Figure 9-1. The Seven Quality Control Tools

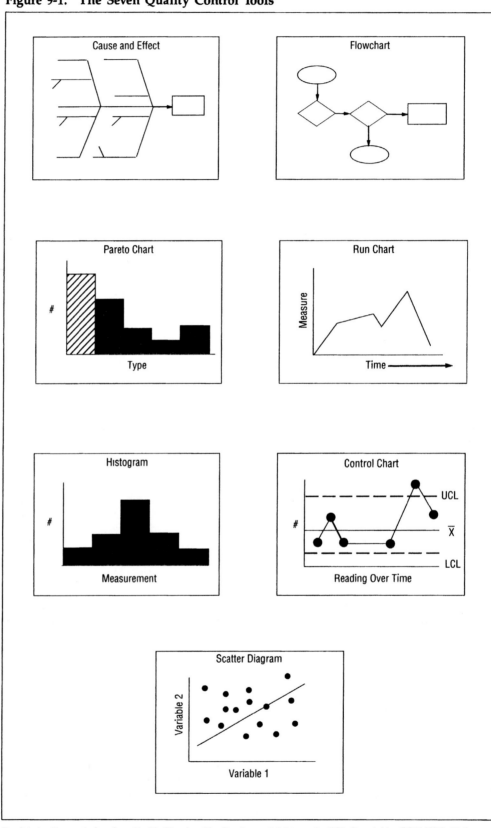

Reprinted, with permission, from *Hoshin Planning: The Developmental Approach*, 1985. Copyright © GOAL/QPC, Methuen, MA 01844.

Figure 9-2. The Seven Management Tools

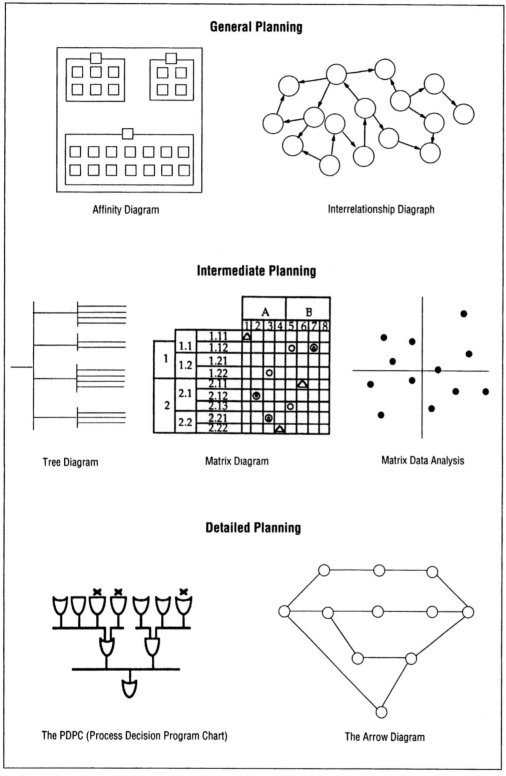

Reprinted, with permission, from *Hoshin Planning: The Developmental Approach*, 1985. Copyright © GOAL/QPC, Methuen, MA 01844.

Rather than surveying all the many existing tools, the following two chapters focus on the most versatile and user-friendly ones currently being used by health care managers. These tools are especially good starters for managers who are relatively new to quality improvement methodology. Also, these tools require no prior knowledge of statistics.

Specifically, this part of the book concentrates on the following tools:

- Tools for collecting and displaying data
  - Focus groups
  - Surveys
  - Check sheets
  - Logs
  - Histograms
  - Pareto charts
  - Trend charts and run charts
- Tools for making improvements
  - Flowcharts
  - Brainstorming
  - Affinity charts
  - Relationships diagrams
  - Cause-and-effect diagrams
  - Force-field analysis
  - Decision matrices
  - Tree diagrams
  - Tools for action planning

Each of these tools will be described in the context of health care quality improvement. The discussion of each includes a description of the tool and its uses, instructions for its development or construction, various examples, and tips and cautions related to its most effective uses.

References

1. Imai, M. *Kaizen: The Key to Japan's Competitive Success.* New York City: Random House, 1986.

2. King, B. *Hoshin Planning: The Developmental Approach.* Methuen, MA: Goal/QPC, 1990, p. 1–13.

3. King, pp. 1-14, 1-15.

Chapter 10

Tools for Collecting and Displaying Data

To what extent are current performance levels meeting customer expectations? How is current performance compared to past performance? Does performance seem to be slipping or improving? How variable or consistent is performance? What are the primary causes of performance problems? Which causes have the most impact? How does performance after you've implemented an improvement plan compare to performance before you implemented your plan? These questions often arise when you pursue improvement opportunities. Your ability to answer these important questions reliably and rationally depends on your ability to collect meaningful information rather than just reams of data.

The Juran Institute's *Quality Improvement Tools*[1] workbook identifies important differences between data and information:

- Data equal facts.
- Information equals answers to questions.
- Information includes data.
- Data do not necessarily include information.

When a problem or improvement opportunity becomes evident, the first step is to clarify the questions surrounding that problem (or opportunity) and determine how to gather useful information that both enlightens your approach to the problem and clearly answers your questions. For example, if your initial problem is that patients and physicians report dissatisfaction with telephone communications with your organization, you would need to decide which calls to study. How do you approach the problem? By department? By unit? Inbound calls? Outbound calls? Times of calls? Nature of calls? Number of rings before answering? You might record information about frequency of occurrence during a certain time period; costs and revenue associated with calls; number of patients served; waiting time; successes versus failures; time taken to accomplish a task; number of people involved; type of errors or problems; and so forth. There are so many possibilities that it is imperative that you clarify your purpose before you can identify the kind of data that will translate into useful information.

The second step is to determine the best way to summarize and communicate the answers to your questions. There are several tools that graphically illustrate the results of data collection so that you and your colleagues can identify at a glance any patterns, trends, and priorities that emerge.

Finally, once you know what questions you are answering and how to show the results, you need to figure out the logistical specifics:

- *Where.* Decide at which points in the process you can collect data to answer your question.
- *When.* Decide your time frame for collecting the data (for example, hours, minutes, dates, weeks, shifts, quarters).
- *Who.* Determine who in the process can provide the data most conveniently without interfering with the process as it currently works.
- *How.* Decide how to gather the data from the people who have it, with minimum interference and probability of error. Design any forms that will be needed to capture the data clearly and simply, labeling columns and rows and leaving plenty of space for data entry.

□ Checks against Bias in Data Collection

Measures should be taken to ensure that the data-collection tactics yield trustworthy data. There are several reasons why data might be untrustworthy:

- *Bias from fear.* Some people are afraid to accurately report what they think is inadequate performance for fear that it will reflect poorly on them. They record data that reflect their preferred reality and thus produce data that don't reflect reality at all.
- *Distraction bias.* Some people are distracted by the process of their responsibilities and forget to record the data. Thus, they guess in order to avoid admitting their oversight.
- *Sampling error.* When you include only a sample of events, it is possible to exclude inadvertently key events or parts of your process. Be sure that your sampling technique leads to collecting data that are representative of all the important times and conditions surrounding the process.
- *Intrusion bias.* The process you use to collect data may very well influence the results you get. For example, when staff know that speed is being measured, they may work beyond their normal speed.
- *Perception bias.* The people collecting the data might have selective perception that colors what they see. As a result, the data might not reflect fact as much as the data collector's own version of reality.
- *Operational bias.* Some data collectors might not follow the procedures you develop because they have not been adequately trained, the procedures are unwieldy, or the collectors are distracted by their other responsibilities.
- *Nonresponse bias.* When staff collecting data do not record *every* bit of data during the defined time period, it is not valid to generalize from this incomplete data set.

Following are several steps you can take to counteract these sources of bias:

- *Make your data-collection devices "face valid."* When people close to the work look at the device you are planning to use, they should be able to see how the data will answer your questions. On the face of it, they see that the data gathered will be trustworthy and meaningful.
- *Select data collectors who you believe can be unbiased.* They should be people who have easy and immediate access to the process you want them to observe and record.

- *Make your forms simple.* They should be so clear that they are almost self-explanatory.
- *Test and refine your forms and instructions.* Debug them with the people who will collect the data; make sure they work.
- *Audit the data-collection process.* Occasionally, check up on data collectors in a non-threatening way. Have multiple collectors record the data simultaneously to determine interrater reliability. If the data vary from one collector to another, work with both people to determine where the discrepancies are and fix the data-collection process to eliminate this variation.

This chapter describes several versatile and user-friendly tools for data collection and display—tools that *inform* your quest to solve problems and make improvements. Figure 10-1 lists these tools and their uses. As indicated in the figure, some can be used to collect data, others to display data, and still others to collect and display data simultaneously.

Figure 10-1. Tools for Data Collection and Display

	Collect Data	Display Data
Focus groups	X	
Surveys	X	
Check sheets	X	
Logs	X	
Histograms	X	X
Pareto charts		X
Trend charts	X	X
Run charts	X	X
Control charts	X	X

☐ Tool 1: Focus Group

The *focus group* is a powerful information-gathering technique that uses small-group discussion to identify the views of people in the group about a certain subject. A facilitator leads the discussion using a question guide. Focus groups work best when questions are open-ended and the facilitator encourages substantial discussion of each question.

The advantage of focus groups over written surveys is that you can probe and follow up for more information. In addition, the discussion tends to achieve depth because the interaction among participants triggers additional thoughts.

Uses of Focus Groups in Quality Improvement

In your efforts to improve quality, focus groups can be used toward six ends:

- To identify requirements and expectations (with customers and staff)
- To solicit perceptions of your area's performance in meeting requirements (with customers, staff, and knowledgeable observers)
- To clarify the dynamics or intricacies of experience or interaction with your area so you can better focus your improvement efforts (with customers, staff, and knowledgeable observers)
- To generate improvement opportunities and ideas (with customers, staff, experts, and knowledgeable observers)
- To field-test changes, solutions, or options in order to refine or select among them (with customers, staff, and experts)
- To develop surveys based on customer expectations (with customers and staff)

Following are some examples of how focus groups have been used:

- A department head identified her customers and held a focus group with representatives from each customer group to identify customer expectations of her area. Using the results, she devised a method of monitoring her area's performance in relation to each expectation.
- The director of pathology identified the primary expectations physicians have of the pathology department. These included rapid turnaround of lab results, accuracy of results, and responsiveness to physician questions and concerns. The director then held a focus group with a few physicians each month to monitor how the department was doing with regard to those particular expectations.
- The vice-president of nursing heard rumblings about staff morale. She sponsored several focus groups with staff to identify the dynamics her staff members perceived as contributing to their quality of work life.
- The director of physical therapy wanted to consider the possibility of creating satellite physical therapy areas on patient units to reduce the need for transporters; encourage a team approach to patients among physicians, nurses, and physical therapists; make services more accessible to patients; and enable patients to wait in their rooms in case of delays. She held focus groups with physicians, nurses, physical therapists, patients, and transporters to field-test the idea and invite their help in clarifying each customer group's expectations.
- The director of nutrition services held a focus group (she called it a user group) with members of each of her department's internal customers (nurses, employees, physicians, and others) to find out about areas of satisfaction and dissatisfaction with her department during the past month.

Procedure

The size of focus groups varies between 5 and 12 individuals. Typically, focus groups last between 60 and 90 minutes. The facilitator can be someone in your department who is a good listener and is viewed as being open-minded, fair, and good with people. This person should also have some experience in leading group discussions and be able to withhold his or her own opinions in favor of encouraging openness and communication among group members. If no such person is available, your organization may have trainers, organizational development specialists, or marketing specialists who could serve as facilitators for you. Frequently, these people are experienced in conducting these kinds of meetings.

Before the Focus Group
In advance of the focus group, it is important to complete the following preparations:

- Find a conducive place for the meeting that is free of distraction and, ideally, has one large table and several chairs.
- Clarify your purpose to the participants ahead of time.
- Prepare a guide that includes open-ended questions that encourage a range of responses and that "probe" for specifics, such as who, what, when, why, and where.
- Test your questions on a nonparticipant and invite reactions and suggestions. Refine the question guide based on your feedback.

During the Focus Group
Although conducting a focus group does not require extensive training, it is important to follow established guidelines, which facilitate the group's understanding of the process and their interaction with each other:

- *Introduce purpose.* Even though you might have described the purpose of the focus group to the participants when you invited them to participate, always begin the session by recapping the purpose of the discussion. Some members may not remember the purpose clearly, others may have different interpretations of it, and so forth. A brief description of the purpose to the whole group at the beginning also serves to focus everyone's attention on the issue to be discussed. For example, "Pharmacy is working to improve the quality of service to its customers. Nursing has been identified as a key customer of the department. In an effort to identify the kind of service that nursing wants and expects from pharmacy, I've been asked to convene a select group of nurses to discuss their expectations of the department so that we can focus our improvement efforts on what matters most to you, our customers."
- *General introductions.* The facilitator introduces himself or herself and asks people to introduce themselves. Go around the room so everyone gets a turn.
- *Establish ground rules.* In order for the discussion to proceed smoothly, participants need to know how and when they are expected to interact. You can pose a question and invite people to respond at random. Or for questions that are particularly crucial, you can go around the group so that every person has a chance to answer. For example, the facilitator might explain the procedure as follows: "Let me explain how this discussion will work. I have some questions I want you to address. After beginning, I'd like you to share your views. I want to give everyone a chance to answer the question if they wish. Please feel free to agree or disagree with one another or say something entirely different. There's no need to make decisions or reach an agreement. I just want to hear what you think.

  "I'm going to tape-record [or take notes on] what's said so that I don't forget. I do want to assure you of confidentiality. I'll summarize what I learn, but I won't name names. The session will last an hour. I want to thank you in advance for participating."
- *Conduct discussion.* The facilitator begins the discussion by asking one of the prepared questions and allowing the participants to respond. He or she will not usually intervene in the discussion until several people have offered their views or unless some points have been raised that need further probing. Following is an example of questions and a chart used for a focus group on pharmacy department service:
  - What do you like about the services provided by the pharmacy department?
  - What do you see as problems in the department's delivery of service?
  - A copy of the chart shown in figure 10-2 was either passed out to the participants or drawn on a flip chart or chalkboard. The chart was then explained to the group. The group was then probed for strengths and weaknesses in each box relevant to the department's area of responsibility.
  - If you ran the department, what would you fix? Any ideas about how?

Figure 10-2. Chart Used in Focus Group to Probe for Department's Strengths and Weaknesses

Key components	When you evaluate this department's services, what do you see as:	
	This department's strengths	This department's weaknesses
Technical/clinical competence		
Environment		
People skills		
Processes/systems/procedures		
Amenities/extras		

- *Facilitator tips.* Following are some suggestions for facilitating the focus group discussion:
  - Throughout, use reflective listening and paraphrasing to make sure you're clear on what people are saying.
  - After one person answers, invite other responses with cues such as "How do other people see this?" or "To what extent do people agree with that?" or "Does anyone see this differently?"
  - Use positive, accepting acknowledgments such as "Uh-huh" and "yes" and nod to encourage people to express themselves.
  - Probe and push but at no time disagree with what someone says.
- *End with appreciation.* Express your appreciation to people for participating. Reiterate the purpose the group was meant to serve. For example, "As I said, we convened this group so we could learn from our key customers what matters to you in terms of our department's service. Now, we'll take what we've learned today and use it to help us pick our department's priorities for service improvement. Thank you all for coming."

After the Focus Group

Summarize what focus group members said as soon as possible before the substance fades. Be descriptive, not interpretive. Ideally, you should write down the dominant themes and prominent points immediately after the session. Later, you should listen to the tape in order to obtain anything that was missed, as well as any quotes that document central themes. Then, present your findings to others who can help you interpret, draw conclusions, and make decisions. Figure 10-3 is an example of a form that might be used to summarize your findings.

User Groups

A variation on the focus group is the *user group,* which is a term used by many to describe a focus group that one department conducts with another department on a regular basis. These are simple and effective customer feedback devices for tapping the perceptions of your internal customers, particularly other departments.

A user group consists of representatives from one of your internal customer groups. You might convene this group every month for an hour or so to ask them the following questions:

- How are we treating you lately?
- You said you expect of us quick turnaround, accuracy, and responsiveness. Looking at these expectations one at a time, I'd like to know how we're doing.
- What changes would you suggest in the way our department operates?

Your role is to listen, listen, listen, so that you do not miss the specifics. Be sure to have someone take notes or tape-record the discussion. Then summarize the results, focusing on user perceptions of your department's degree of success on quality or service attributes that matter to them. Share the results with your staff without being punitive. Use the results to celebrate excellent performance and redirect your improvement priorities.

Figure 10-3. Example of Form to Summarize Focus Group Results

Customer Group: Physicians*			
Systems/Procedures That Work Well for Our Physicians	The Specific Strengths	Systems That Our Physicians Find Unfriendly	Their Specific Observations and Frustrations
Chart retrieval postdischarge	Helpful staff Quick location of charts	Admissions from ER to inpatient beds	Takes too long Patient not kept informed
Valet parking	Rapid access to car Convenience	Turnaround of lab results	Lost results Slow turnaround Results not on charts
Utilization review of diagnosis	Length-of-stay guidelines helpful	Nuclear medicine	Results not on charts No feedback
Social services' early involvement in discharge planning	Physician input honored Discharge support planned in time	Information entry on patient charts	Lost information Delays Incomplete

*You received many complaints from physicians about systems in your department that are not customer-friendly. You hold a focus group for physicians to find out the specifics so you can target improvement opportunities. You summarize the results on a chart like this one.

□ Tool 2: Surveys

For the purposes of this discussion, *surveys* are written questionnaires used to collect quantitative data. They elicit perceptions at one point in time. Each question takes a snapshot of one element of performance, which you can compare to another snapshot when you survey at a later point. Surveys are quantitative devices for collecting feedback to enlighten decision making. They are particularly useful for soliciting perceptions of service from customers when you want to identify reliable trends and patterns for large numbers of people in an efficient manner.

You can distribute surveys by mail or hand them out at the last point in your interactions with customers. Or you can use them as formats for face-to-face or telephone interviews.

Uses of Surveys in Quality Improvement

Surveys can be used in the following ways:

- To identify customer or staff expectations and needs. You can ask customers to express the relative importance they place on various attributes of your service so that you know their primary criteria for evaluating your service, which are the contributors to their satisfaction.
- To monitor customer satisfaction with the attributes of your service that are important to them. Survey results can easily be visualized on trend charts that show, for example, "percent negative ratings" or "percent excellent ratings." You can use these to communicate results to staff.
- To identify the gap or discrepancy between *real* and *desired* performance in order to target problems or improvement opportunities. A Pareto chart (described later in this chapter) can be used to identify high-priority problems from survey results.
- To measure the effects of an improvement to see whether customer or staff perceptions improved as a result of it.
- To elicit reactions to hypothetical improvement alternatives.
- To tune your staff in to their customers, firsthand if you have staff serve as data collectors and analyzers.
- To show your customers or staff that you care what they think.

How to Develop and Conduct a Survey

Following are the basic steps to follow in developing and implementing a survey:

1. *Clarify the purposes of your survey.* What exactly do you want to find out? The percentage of satisfied patients? The service attribute most important to a large number of people? The relative strengths and weaknesses of your department on various quality or service dimensions?
2. *Clarify whom you want to survey—the respondents.* All patients, every day? A 20 percent sample of patients each month? A 20 percent sample of patients at randomly selected times in order to cover all three shifts? Make these decisions first on "face validity" or common sense. A good guideline is to survey a minimum of 30 people of each type you want to include in order to secure a pattern of results. You might consult your marketing department for advice on the appropriate sample size for your particular study.
3. *Design questions in line with your purposes.* It helps to brainstorm possibilities with a group of people who understand your purpose. Then refine the questions and try them out on your group for clarity and purposefulness.
4. *Convene people who are representative of the group you want to survey.* Using a focus group format, involve them in fine-tuning the questions. Try out the questions you want to ask and refine them. Use the feedback to revise the questions so that they are clear, understandable, and unbiased from the perspective of your respondents and from your perspective so that they generate useful information.
5. *Given your resources, determine how to survey people so that you will have confidence in the results.* How often? By whom? Using what means? For example, will you distribute a paper-and-pencil survey? If so, will you mail it, or will a staff member personally deliver it to respondents and ask for their cooperation? Or, if patients are too ill or might have difficulty reading the survey, will you consider having staff members trained as interviewers administer the survey in person or by phone? There are no hard-and-fast rules about how to make these decisions. You need to talk with your team and determine what is feasible and what you can defend as a trustworthy technique.
6. *Standardize the survey process—the introduction, the words to be used, and the conditions under which respondents complete the surveys.* If you do not standardize these factors, you will find yourself administering different instruments and getting results that are not comparable.

7. *Train the people involved in survey distribution and data collection.* Set up a meeting to orient the data collectors to the purposes and methods involved in the survey. Demonstrate how to conduct the survey and emphasize the need for everyone to administer the survey the same way for the sake of reliable results. Give people a chance to practice with supervision and feedback. Make sure they master the survey explanation and technique.

Following are some examples of survey instruments used by different departments:

- A short *service report card* is shown in figure 10-4. This was used by an admitting department to survey one of its customer groups, physicians' office managers.
- The instrument shown in figure 10-5 was designed by a pharmacy department to monitor its service to nurses, its primary internal customers. To establish the questions, pharmacy staff interviewed nurses about their priorities regarding service from the pharmacy.
- A survey developed by a nursing–pharmacy improvement team is shown in figure 10-6. This survey was used to collect information about patients' perceptions of service related to medications.
- At a psychiatric center, department directors interviewed their internal customers to identify service attributes important to them and then surveyed these customers periodically to monitor satisfaction levels and identify problems. Figure 10-7 (p. 113) shows the questionnaires used for these periodic surveys.

Figure 10-4. "Service Report Card" Survey

Dear Office Manager,

Our Admitting Department wants to do its part in making it easy for you to meet your patients' needs in our hospital. Will you please help by completing and returning the attached "Service Report Card" that asks you to evaluate our services? The card is already addressed and stamped for your convenience. Thank you very much.

1. *Courtesy:* When you call Admitting, how courteous are the people who handle your calls?

    very rude   1   2   3   4   very courteous

2. *Speed:* When you call Admitting, how quickly do we meet your needs?

    very slowly   1   2   3   4   very quickly

3. *Follow-through:* When people in Admitting tell you they'll get back to you about something (e.g., with information, an answer to your question, etc.), how likely are they to follow through as promised?

    not likely at all   1   2   3   4   very likely

4. *Competence:* When you deal with our department, how competent are staff in meeting your needs?

    very incompetent   1   2   3   4   very competent

5. *How do we compare to other hospitals?* If you admit patients to other hospitals, how do you rate our department's effectiveness in meeting your needs—compared to departments in other hospitals?

    much worse   1   2   3   4   much better

6. What is your biggest frustration with our department?

7. Please add any further comments and suggestions.

Thank you.

• Radiology department members identified patients' expectations of their department at each step in their service cycle. Then, each week, they focused on one step in the cycle and surveyed customers about their satisfaction with performance at that step. Figure 10-8 (p. 115) shows the simple spot survey they used on an intermittent schedule to monitor patients' perceptions of technologists' performance.

Figure 10-5. Pharmacy Department Survey Instrument to Monitor Its Service to Nursing

1. In filling routine orders, the Pharmacy is	1	2	3	4
	timely			untimely
2. In filling STAT orders, the Pharmacy is	1	2	3	4
	quick to respond			slow to respond
3. The attitude of Pharmacy personnel is	1	2	3	4
	professional			unprofessional
4. Drug information supplied by the Pharmacy is	1	2	3	4
	useful			not useful
5. The Pharmacy's response to changing needs is	1	2	3	4
	appropriate			inappropriate
6. The hours of Pharmacy coverage are	1	2	3	4
	adequate			inadequate
7. The procedures to use Pharmacy services are	1	2	3	4
	efficient			cumbersome

Reprinted, with permission, from the Einstein Consulting Group, Philadelphia, 1989.

Figure 10-6. Survey Instrument to Monitor Patient Perception of Medication Service

Will You Help Us Improve Our Services?

Our pharmacy and nursing departments work together to provide you with the medication you need while you're under our care. These two departments are currently working together to enhance their service and solve any problems that patients are having with medication.

Will you please help by sharing your experience with us?

1. Have you had any problems with your medications while you've been here? Please describe:

2. Have medications been:

	often			rarely
Delivered on time?	1	2	3	4
Explained to you?	1	2	3	4
Correct item?	1	2	3	4
Given courteously?	1	2	3	4
Available when needed?	1	2	3	4

3. How can we improve our services related to medications?

Your responses will be kept strictly confidential. Please leave this completed form on your meal tray. Your response will be very helpful to us. Thank you very much.

Reprinted, with permission, from Albert Einstein Healthcare Foundation, 1990.

Figure 10-7. Internal Customer Survey: Psychiatric Hospital's Rating of Different Departments

A. Center Nursing Unit

1. The unit interacts with other departments with

    1   2   3   4
    respect   aloofness

2. The unit follows other departments' applicable procedures

    1   2   3   4
    cooperatively   uncooperatively

3. The unit responds to other departments' requests

    1   2   3   4
    quickly   reluctantly

4. The operation of the unit on day shift appears

    1   2   3   4
    organized   disorganized

    on evening shift appears

    1   2   3   4
    organized   disorganized

    on night shift appears

    1   2   3   4
    organized   disorganized

    on all weekend shifts appears

    1   2   3   4
    organized   disorganized

5. When there are interdepartmental problems, the staff approaches resolutions as

    1   2   3   4
    team members   dictators

6. The perception of care on this unit is

    1   2   3   4
    excellent   poor

7. Communication to other departments of changes on the unit that affect them is

    1   2   3   4
    timely   after the fact

8. Communication to other departments about changes on the unit that affect them is

    1   2   3   4
    clear   unclear

9. Unit personnel usually project attitudes that are

    1   2   3   4
    positive   negative

10. Care and concern for the patients appear to be

    1   2   3   4
    primary   an afterthought

11. When it comes to sensitivity to patients, the staff's performance is

    1   2   3   4
    excellent   poor

B. Dietary

1. The cafeteria environment is

    1   2   3   4
    comfortable   uncomfortable

2. The variety on the menu is

    1   2   3   4
    very good   poor

3. Cafeteria services are provided

    1   2   3   4
    efficiently   inefficiently

4. Monthly cafeteria specials are

    1   2   3   4
    wonderful   awful

5. The staff is courteous and helpful

    1   2   3   4
    consistently   inconsistently

6. The cleanliness of dishes and serviceware is

    1   2   3   4
    excellent   poor

7. Therapeutic visitation to the patient is

    1   2   3   4
    timely   untimely

8. Special functions are done with imagination

    1   2   3   4
    routinely   sporadically

(continued on next page)

Figure 10-7. (Continued)

9. Communication between dietary and other departments is

    1   2   3   4
    open   restrained

10. Criticism and suggestions are accepted

    1   2   3   4
    readily   reluctantly

C. Diagnostic Services

In measuring turnaround time in performing the test and returning the results:

1. The EKG service is

    1   2   3   4
    prompt   too slow

2. The EEG service is

    1   2   3   4
    prompt   too slow

3. The ECT service is

    1   2   3   4
    prompt   too slow

4. The laboratory service is

    1   2   3   4
    prompt   too slow

5. The radiology service is

    1   2   3   4
    prompt   too slow

6. The CT scanning service is

    1   2   3   4
    prompt   too slow

D. Business Office

1. When bills are prepared for patients or insurance carriers, the information is

    1   2   3   4
    accurate   inaccurate

2. When bills are prepared for patients or insurance carriers, the information is

    1   2   3   4
    timely   slow

3. Personnel are

    1   2   3   4
    courteous   rude

4. Personnel are

    1   2   3   4
    responsive   unresponsive

E. Purchasing

1. In an emergency, purchasing is

    1   2   3   4
    responsive   unresponsive

2. Turnaround time from initial paperwork to receipt of order is

    1   2   3   4
    timely   too long

3. Our understanding of the purchasing process, i.e., paperwork, corporate interface is

    1   2   3   4
    very good   needs refreshing

4. Inquiries about purchasing are handled

    1   2   3   4
    quickly   slowly

F. Central Supply

1. Routine turnaround of orders is

    1   2   3   4
    timely   too slow

2. Emergency response to orders is

    1   2   3   4
    prompt   too slow

3. Stock levels are

    1   2   3   4
    appropriate   inappropriate

4. The clerk is generally

    1   2   3   4
    responsive   unresponsive

Reprinted, with permission, from the Philadelphia Psychiatric Center, Philadelphia, 1988.

Figure 10-8. Simple Spot Survey of Technologist's Performance

Will you please help us improve our service in Radiology by answering these quick questions?

How would you rate the behavior of the technologist who performed your procedures?	Very rude		Very courteous	
	1	2	3	4
	Explained procedure poorly/not at all		Explained procedure thoroughly and well	
	1	2	3	4
	Handled me very roughly		Handled me very gently	
	1	2	3	4

Other comments (and please feel free to complain so we know what to fix!):

Please drop in the Survey Box, ask your transporter to drop it in for you, or ask your nurse to drop it in the in-house mail. Thank you so much for your help.

Reprinted, with permission, from Albert Einstein Healthcare Foundation, 1990.

Tips

Following are two important tips in designing and planning your surveys:

1. *Consult your customers.* Too often, surveys are written and used without consulting customers. As a result, people ask questions about quality attributes they *think* are important to customers but may not be. Consultations with customers should be built into the survey design process to determine what is important to customers so that you can ask the right questions. Your survey should also be tested on customers to iron out the kinks and make it easy to read, understand, and answer.
2. *Develop good survey questions.* Good questions are essential to the success of your survey and the following guidelines may be used to formulate them:
   - *The good survey question is clear, easy to read, and easy to understand.* It is user-friendly as determined by respondents.
   - *The good survey question gives the respondent a range of possible responses.* Questions that require a yes–no type of answer do not usually provide helpful information because they force people to choose extreme answers that might not reflect their true opinions. For example, if you asked, "Were nurses courteous?" many people might say yes because some of the nurses were courteous and the respondents would not want those nurses to think they weren't appreciated even though other nurses were rude.

     It is helpful to give respondents four to six choices. More than six is unnecessary and misleading because most people cannot make that many distinctions. Fewer than four choices gives too narrow a set of possibilities and forces people to make judgments they may not feel comfortable with. Some people recommend against an odd number of choices because noncommittal people often pick the middle alternative. When you give an even number of choices, people have to decide whether they lean in one direction or another. As a result, you learn more.

- *The good survey question is unbiased.* Consider this example: How tasty was the food?

  Horrible

  So-so

  Tasty

  Delectable

  This scale is lopsided. Two of the alternatives are clearly on the positive side of the continuum; only one is on the negative side, and one (so-so) is usually considered to be a moderate or noncommittal response. It would be better to replace "so-so" with "tasteless."

- *The scale used for each question must be balanced.* In other words, the values at the highest and lowest ends must be of equal intensity. For example, the following is unbalanced:

  Never   Often

     1   2   3   4

  These values are not balanced; it would be better to offer "rarely" in opposition to "often."

- *Only real possibilities should be included in your scales.* Avoid words such as *never* and *always* as the ends of your scales. In life, *never* and *always* are rare no matter what you are talking about. As a result, when you use these words in survey scales, you render two of your alternatives largely useless.

- *Measure only one attribute in each question.* If you ask, "How courteous and friendly was the receptionist?" you are asking two different questions in one. Consequently, you will not know which attribute triggered the scores you get. If you want to know about both friendliness and courtesy, for example, you need to develop a separate question to measure each attribute.

- *Beware of survey overkill.* Now that health care organizations are becoming more concerned with customer perceptions, there is a risk of surveying the same customers again and again with various types of surveys. You can avoid overkill by doing the following:

  - Coordinate your survey plans with other people who might be conducting surveys to make sure that the same people are not being asked to complete 10 different surveys by 10 different departments. In one hospital, every department with patients as customers was surveying patients. They handled it this way: Admissions surveyed people whose names began with A through C; transport surveyed people whose names began with E through G; and so forth. Intermittently, the departments switched letters.

  - Keep your surveys short. Track your department's performance on a few attributes at a time.

  - Use internal measures other than surveys to monitor your performance. If you know what your customers want, you can translate their expectations into operational requirements and monitor your own performance without having to ask your customers whether they are getting what they want. If they want timely service and *timely* means "within 20 minutes," you can regularly use time charts to track your performance and only occasionally ask customers how timely the service was.

- *Use available resources to help you.* If your organization has marketing professionals, they might be able to help you to develop and test survey questions and even administer the surveys for you.

- *Involve your staff.* This tip is controversial. Research experts tell you to make data collection "unobtrusive." They recommend against using your own people to collect survey data for fear of bias and for fear that "knowing the questions" will influence the results. Depending on your purposes, it might sometimes be wise to defy this advice. If your goal is to satisfy your customers, it will indeed raise your staff's awareness of the important questions when you have your staff collect the data. Often, the more aware they are of the test questions, the more likely they are to perform well so that they can see high scores on the test. The point is that engaging your staff to know the survey questions, interact with customers to collect the data, analyze the data, and see the results is in itself a very powerful intervention that positively improves staff performance. In some cases, staff involvement at the expense of data purity may be worth it.

☐ Tool 3: Check Sheets

A *check sheet* is a form designed to make it easy to record data. It is usually in the format of a diagram or table. All you have to do is place a check or tally mark to reflect an observation, action, or instance of what you are observing. A check sheet enables you to count the frequency of an event or action within specified time periods. It enables you to record these facts in a systematic way as they happen, waiting until later to summarize results, extract patterns, or draw conclusions.

For example, check sheets can be used to track the following:

- The number of nurses absent during different shifts on different days
- The nature of clinic visits
- The incidence of wheelchair requests per time period
- The number of complications associated with each of several diagnoses
- The number of complaints per day of week or by type
- The number of charts signed by each physician within a specific time period
- The demand for certain inventory items and the number of unfulfilled requests per time period
- The number of failed inspections by housekeeping supervisors

Figure 10-9 illustrates one sample check sheet format and four typical check sheets that track complaints by type, tally reasons for rejected bills, tally surgical kit requests by physicians, and track employee absences by day of week. A check sheet designed to identify the kinds of information typically missing from patient charts is shown in figure 10-10 (p. 119).

Check sheets can be used for a variety of purposes. For example:

- *To trigger discussion of performance.* Once you total results, you can discuss the trends, the frequencies of key events, and the distribution or spread of the data that might suggest theories about causes.
- *To search for key causes.* Structured well in advance, check sheets can reveal how people, equipment, methods, and materials influence a problem.
- *To measure the results of a solution or improvement.* Like other measurement tools, check sheets can be used to check up on the results of improvements.
- *Ongoing monitoring.* To keep a tight rein on conformance to your desired process, you can use check sheets to monitor performance, ensuring that you hold your gains and checking that previous problems do not reappear.

Figure 10-9. Five Sample Check Sheets

A. Example Format for Check Sheet

Problem	Hours/Day/Month/Week					Total
	1	2	3	4	5	
1						
2						
3						
4						
Totals						

B. Check Sheet Used to Track Complaints, by Type

Complaint Type	Incidence of Complaints											
	Jan.	Feb.	Mar.	Apr.	May	June	Jul.	Aug.	Sept.	Oct.	Nov.	Dec.
Billing mistake												
Late meal												
Rude staff												
Broken equipment												
Totals												

C. Check Sheet Designed to Tally the Reasons for Rejected Bills

Reason	February			Total
	Outpatient	Inpatient	Emergency Room	
Illegible				
Ineligible person				
Incomplete information				
Unreimbursable charge				
Totals				

D. Check Sheet Designed to Tally Surgical Kits Requested, by Type

	Surgical Kit Requests by Physician					Total
	Week 1	Week 2	Week 3	Week 4	Week 5	
Type 1						
Type 2						
Type 3						
Type 4						
Totals						

E. Check Sheet to Track Employee Absence, by Work Group

Work Group	Employee Absences by Day of Week						
	Mon.	Tues.	Wed.	Thurs.	Fri.	Sat.	Sun.
A							
B							
C							
D							
Totals							

Figure 10-10. Weekly Check Sheet of Information Missing from Charts

Collector: Martin								Week ending: 9/9

Information	Nursing Unit							
	1A	1B	1C	1D	2A	2B	2C	Total
Preadmission tests								
Radiology reports								
Lab results								
Nuclear medicine results								
Medication charges								
Discharge plan								
Totals								

□ Tool 4: Logs

Logs are simple chronological records or diaries that track the sequence of events, the nature of errors or complaints, and the times they occur. Logs must be translated into a summary format in order to reveal their meaning or the patterns within the recorded data. Figure 10-11 shows a log used by a receptionist to track outpatient waiting times and the summary chart that was derived from it. Examples of a complaint log and a medication error log are shown in figures 10-12 and 10-13, respectively.

How to Develop a Log

Following are the steps that should be taken in developing logs:

1. Determine the key elements needed to define what you want to record (for example, time, place, content, people responsible, and so forth).
2. Set up a chart with these elements as column titles.
3. Train staff at the point of observation to record the appropriate information in each column.
4. Develop a format for synthesizing and summarizing the data recorded in the log (for example, a histogram, tally sheets by category, and the like).

Tips

The following two tips are useful in planning and designing a log:

1. Keep logging simple; make sure the staff members recording the data record only the raw data without seeking to identify or extract patterns. At periodic intervals, use a tally sheet, histogram, or Pareto chart to show the patterns in the raw data.
2. Engage your staff in developing the log format because logs must be easy to complete and user-friendly.

Figure 10-11. Log to Track Outpatient Waiting Time and Summary of Results

Log				
Patient Name	**Provider**	**Arrival Time**	**Time Taken for Appointment**	**Wait Time**

Summary of Log Results (in minutes)								
	0–10	**11–20**	**21–30**	**31–40**	**41–50**	**51–60**	**71–80**	**81+**
# of patients waiting								
% of patients								

Figure 10-12. Example of Complaint Log

Date: March 16, 1991   Shift 1 2 3   Unit 3W

Time	Complainer	Complaint	Staff Acting	Action Taken	Response Time
11:30	Smith	Unchanged linen	H.S.	Call linen	2 hrs., 20 min.
12:15	Harper	No pain meds. delivery	M.L.	Call pharmacy	45 min.
1:30	Smith	Still no changed linen	H.S.	Call linen	20 more min.
2:10	Morgan	"Inedible" food	M.L.	Call nutritionist	1 hr.

Figure 10-13. Example of Medication Error Log

Medication Errors
Date: _____

Error Described	Whose Error?	Detected How	Action to Take
Dosage error	Pharmacy	Quality check	Correct it; tell supervisor
Late delivery	Nursing	Patient complaint	Deliver to patient
Pills, not liquid as requested	Medical secretary	Patient complaint	Stat order to pharmacy
Dosage error	Physician	Pharmacy doctor	Pharmacy calls
Wrong strength	Pharmacy	Quality check	Nursing calls pharmacy supervisor

□ Tool 5: Histograms

A *histogram* is a bar graph that shows, in easy-to-read pictorial form, the distribution of data points related to some measurable characteristic. However, before we explore the pictorial display of data provided in a histogram, it may be useful to review some important information about the classification of data, which should help illuminate the intuitive meaning in a histogram.

Dealing with Data

Consider the data shown in figure 10-14. As you examine these data, you will find it difficult to tell at a glance how they are distributed. Looking closely at the raw data (section A of figure 10-14), you'll notice that the lowest number is 25 and the highest is 90. But other than that, there is little you can tell about the data points by simply looking at them.

Figure 10-14. Random Samples of 50 Laboratory Turnaround Times for Glucose (minutes)

A. Raw Data

25	42	52	85	32
75	32	36	28	36
50	27	32	32	25
40	48	29	39	29
30	36	55	29	56
60	50	28	31	68
28	90	32	49	72
32	27	40	50	85
49	25	39	28	30
86	44	38	30	28

B. Arrayed Data

25	29	32	40	55
25	29	32	42	56
25	29	32	44	60
27	30	36	48	68
27	30	36	49	72
28	30	36	49	75
28	31	38	50	85
28	32	39	50	85
28	32	39	50	86
28	32	40	52	90

C. Data Classified into Intervals

Class	Class Limits	Class Frequency
1	25–31	17
2	32–38	10
3	39–45	6
4	46–52	7
5	53–59	2
6	60–66	1
7	67–73	2
8	74–80	1
9	81–87	3
10	88–94	1

The way to see these data more clearly is to make an array. In an array, the numbers are arranged from lowest to highest (section B of figure 10-14). The array shows that fewer than half of the turnaround times are 30 minutes or less and that only a few exceed 75 minutes. However, the data are still difficult to understand.

One way to compress the data is to classify them into equal intervals (section C of figure 10-14). Experts recommend between 6 and 20 intervals. More than 20 intervals are difficult to manipulate and fewer than 6 may result in information being lost among the data.

To decide on the number, it helps to look at the data. The data points in figure 10-14 range from 25 to 90. When you subtract 25 from 90, you find a range of 65. If you were to divide these data into 10 intervals, the width of each would be 6.5 per interval. For this example, it makes sense to use 10 intervals, each 7 minutes long. The number of intervals, the width of each, and the upper and lower boundaries are arbitrary, but they should allow for easy accessibility of information. Interval boundaries should be carefully defined so that they do not overlap. For example, the boundaries might look like this: 1–10, 11–20, 21–30, and so on. The number of observations in any interval is called the frequency and is denoted by the symbol f.

Returning to the example, for each class, or interval, we see its boundaries, or limits, and the frequency, or count, of data points within each. The data now begin to provide meaningful information. However, a graphic display will make the patterns and characteristics stand out even more.

A common method for dealing with a mass of data, the histogram helps to display the data in manageable form. It is a bar graph without spaces between the bars because the data are in continuous intervals. Figure 10-15 shows a histogram displaying the data introduced in figure 10-14. As you can see, the data have now been made even more accessible.

Case Example

After flowcharting the process of triage in a hospital's emergency department, an improvement team wanted to analyze the time it took for a patient to go through the triage process

Figure 10-15. Example of Histogram for Laboratory Turnaround Time

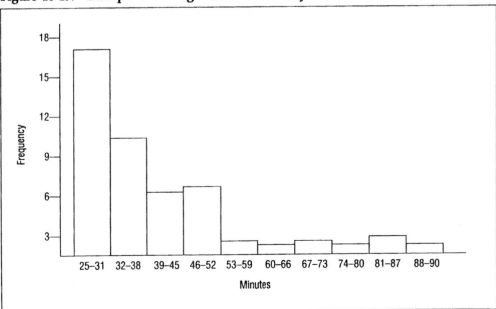

and arrive in the minor treatment area. Every day for a month, the following data for each patient were recorded in a log:

- Time of arrival
- Time patient was greeted by a nurse
- Time patient was completely evaluated by the nurse and documentation was completed
- Time patient was sent to registration
- Time registration was completed
- Time patient was placed in a treatment room

These times for each patient were entered into a computer program (in this case, Lotus™). The team calculated the time interval and the average time (in minutes) for each activity for a representative sample of patients, as follows:

Arrival to greeting	5
Greeting to evaluation completed	15
Evaluation completed to registration	10
Time to register	12
Time from registration to patient placed in treatment room	10
Total triage time	52

The team chose to focus on registration time. Team members analyzed the data for registration times using a score sheet to find the frequency distribution of the various times it took to register patients (see figure 10-16). You can see a pattern developing as the tallying occurs. This pattern becomes even clearer in the histogram shown in figure 10-17.

The team then decided to focus on a time frame of 15 to 19 minutes. The histogram results were used to generate questions. The first question was: "Was there any consistency regarding the time of day of registration times taking from 15 to 19 minutes?" (*Note:* If you use computers to analyze data, be sure to collect the data in military time: 0 to 24 hours. The team forgot to do this and had to reenter all the data.)

Team members asked the computer to find the records for 100 patients in the 15-to-19-minute time frame. They then arranged the data according to time of day by number of occurrences to determine whether patterns existed. The results are shown in figures 10-18 and 10-19. The team was than able to focus attention on the time frame of 16:00 to 19:59.

Figure 10-16. Score Sheet Showing Frequency Distribution of Emergency Department Triage Registration Times

Registration Times	Number of Patients
25-30 ⅬⅢⅠ ⅬⅢⅠ ⅬⅢⅠ	15
20-24 ⅬⅢⅠ ⅬⅢⅠ ⅬⅢⅠ . . .	45
15-19 ⅬⅢⅠ ⅬⅢⅠ ⅬⅢⅠ . . .	100
10-14 ⅬⅢⅠ ⅬⅢⅠ ⅬⅢⅠ . . .	200
5-9 ⅬⅢⅠ ⅬⅢⅠ ⅬⅢⅠ . . .	40
0-4	0

Figure 10-17. Histogram of Data in Figure 10-16

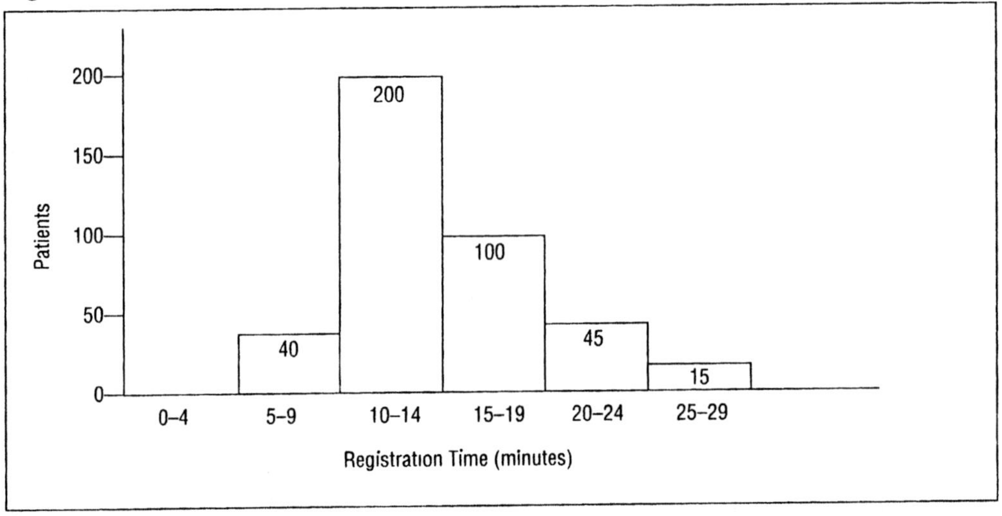

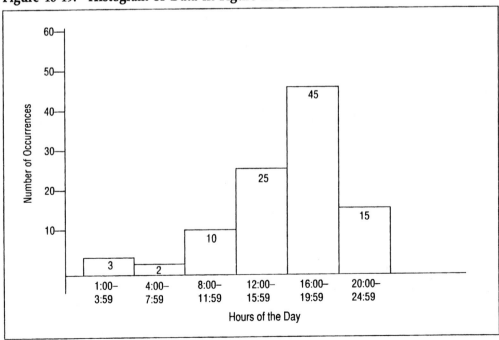

Figure 10-18. Data for 100 Patients, Arrayed by Time of Day and Number of Occurrences

Hours of the Day	Total Patients
1:00 - 3:59	3
4:00 - 7:59	2
8:00 - 11:59	10
12:00 - 15:59	25
16:00 - 19:59	45
20:00 - 24:59	15
	100

Figure 10-19. Histogram of Data in Figure 10-18

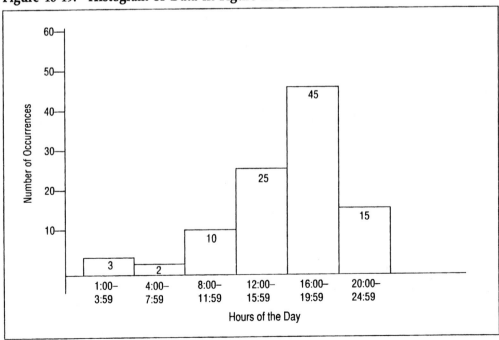

To summarize, presenting data in a histogram helps to provide a clear picture of the problem or the components of the problem. The following describes characteristics of a histogram:

- It is the simplest graphic representation of data.
- It must be used with continuous data, which can be either interval or ratio data.
- Class intervals cannot overlap.
- Class intervals are depicted on the horizontal line, and the frequency data (number of occurrences) are displayed on the vertical axis.

The Nuts and Bolts of Histograms

All repeated events or processes vary in the results they produce over time. The degree and nature of this variation helps you to generate theories about problems in your process, the conditions under which your problem is most severe, and how you might focus your efforts to improve the process. A histogram visually communicates information about variation in a process in a way that helps you to generate questions that focus your improvement efforts. After you create the histogram, you need to revisit your process to answer the questions the histogram raises.

Technically, a histogram consists of a series of equal-width columns, or bars, of differing heights, as shown in figure 10-20. The width of each column represents a preset interval, or class, within the total range of data, or observations. However, the height of each column varies because each column reflects the number of data points or observations within that class or interval.

Interpretations

When observing natural data, it is typical to see many observations piling up toward the middle, which reflects the central tendency of the bell-shaped (normal) curve. As you move away from the center, you see progressively fewer data points. Sometimes, the histogram does not show a normal distribution around a central tendency. Instead, it might show a different pattern of variation that can give important clues about the dynamics of your problem. Figure 10-21 shows four variations of distribution. Twin peaks,

Figure 10-20. Example of Typical Histogram with Central Tendency Distribution

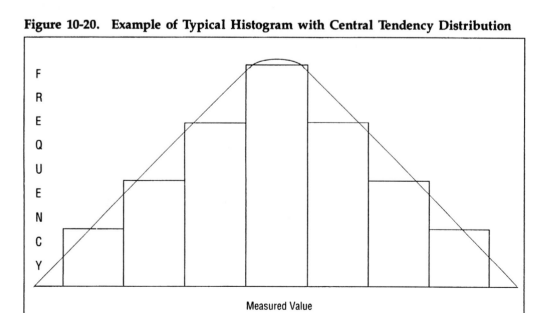

Figure 10-21. Different Histogram Distributions

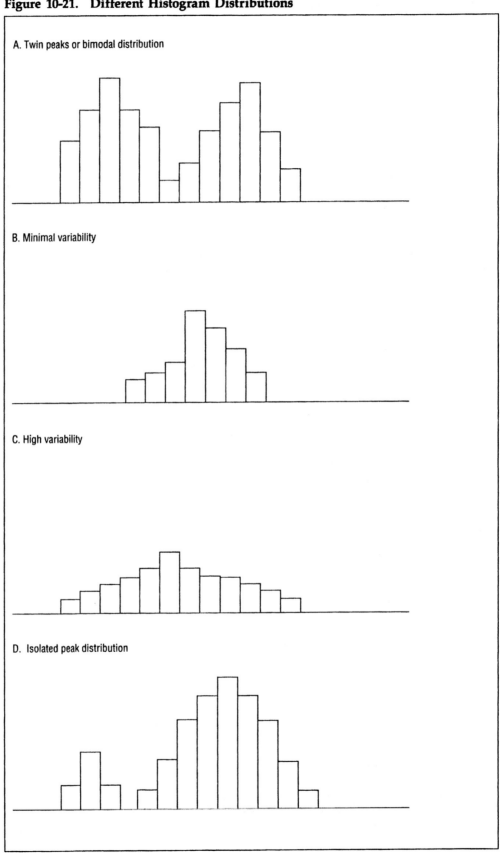

A. Twin peaks or bimodal distribution

B. Minimal variability

C. High variability

D. Isolated peak distribution

or a bimodal, distribution (see section A of figure 10-21) indicates that your data stem from two different operations (for example, shifts, units, work groups, machines). A process producing minimal variability or a narrow range of performance is shown in section B of figure 10-21, and high variability or a wide range of performance is shown in section C.

Some processes are skewed or lopsided, rather than reflecting a bell-shaped curve. The peak is off center because the distribution declines sharply on one side. This occurs because some processes have practical limits with not as many values on both sides of the range. For example, patients cannot be seen in less than zero minutes, and so the left side of the range has a practical limit. The laboratory turnaround time histogram (see figure 10-15) is an example of a skewed histogram. On the other side of the range, however, patients can be kept waiting an infinite period of time. If your histogram reflects this, you need to ask yourself whether this skewed distribution makes logical sense as an inevitable result of the process. If it doesn't, you should become suspicious and search for an explanation. For example, a long tail often reveals customer dissatisfaction, as in long waiting times, or it creates havoc for customers downstream. Because a good process is "in control," extreme variation signals an out-of-control process for which you should seek root causes.

The isolated peak distribution is shown in section D of figure 10-21. In this distribution, a small group of data points is separated from the larger pattern. This suggests that two processes are occurring, not one. The causes of this abnormality should be sought.

As previously indicated, the pattern demonstrated by a histogram has an underlying explanation, which is key to identifying root causes that, when tackled, will improve the performance of and reduce the variation in your process.

Construction

The following eight steps should be used to construct a histogram:

1. Collect the data; count the total number of observations or data points.
2. Arrange the data points in ascending order.
3. Establish the range of your data by subtracting the smallest data point from the largest.
4. Figure out the number of columns you want in your histogram. A minimum of 6 and a maximum of 20 are recommended. Divide the range into this number of columns to establish the width of each interval or class.
5. Write the intervals or classes along the horizontal, or x, axis. Write the frequency scale (numbers or percentages) along the vertical, or y, axis.
6. For each interval or class, then draw a bar that peaks at the number or percentage of data points within that interval or class.
7. Carefully label each axis, title the histogram, and in a box at the side indicate who collected the data and over what time frame.
8. Provide some simple mathematical analysis; calculate the average (mean) and the range, and note them on your graph.

The following questions might be asked to help you follow up on your histogram:

- What is the current level of performance?
- What is the pattern of variation around the current level?
- What are the consequences of this variation?
- What clues does this pattern of variation give you about the scope and nature of your problem? What questions does it raise that you need to investigate? What theories do you now need to test further?

127

Uses

Histograms are generally used for the following two purposes:

1. To understand the variability built into a process so that you can assess the capability of that process to yield acceptable results consistently.
2. To help you generate *alternative* theories about the dynamics of your process and the causes of problems, theories that you then need to confirm or disconfirm through additional observations or analysis.

Precautions

Note the following precautions in the use of histograms:

- Only draw conclusions from histograms drawn from a large sample (40 data points minimum is suggested). Make sure that your data represent the typical and current conditions related to your process. Old data and data influenced by irregular collection procedures throw your conclusions off course.
- It is important to push for alternative explanations of the variation shown in a histogram instead of accepting the first explanation that seems reasonable. People are often misled by sticking to their first hunch about what might explain a pattern when, in fact, they need to take steps to verify their explanation by gathering additional information.

☐ Tool 6: Pareto Charts

Vilfredo Pareto, a 19th-century European economist, depicted in a graph the unequal distribution of wealth among different social classes. He showed that 20 percent of the people have 80 percent of the wealth. His graph became famous and its underlying concept became known as the Pareto principle. Simply stated, 80 percent of the effect is attributable to 20 percent of the causes. The Pareto principle has since become known as the 80–20 rule.

In health care, examples might look like the following:

- Eighty percent of the errors are made by 20 percent of the staff.
- Eighty percent of patient complaints relate to 20 percent of the problems.
- Eighty percent of the long waits in outpatient services are caused by 20 percent of the steps involved in serving outpatients.
- Eighty percent of the equipment breakdowns involve only 20 percent of the equipment.
- Eighty percent of the dissatisfied patients are served on 20 percent of the nursing units.
- Eighty percent of the inappropriate admissions are performed by 20 percent of the referring physicians.
- Eighty percent of the resistance to a quality improvement strategy comes from 20 percent of the staff.
- Eighty percent of the improvements are made by 20 percent of your staff.

The Pareto chart depicts the principle graphically by separating data according to their significance or relative impact.

The Pareto chart is a vertical bar graph, or column graph, that displays the relative importance of the problems or causes you have identified. In actuality, it is a cumulative percentage histogram. It shows individual elements or causes as a percentage of the total, in declining order. The most important or influential problems or causes are represented by the tallest bars on the left of the chart (see figure 10-22). The goal is to focus your attention on the "vital few" in contrast to the "trivial many." Because your time is precious and you cannot tackle all problems or root causes at once, you need to select problems or root causes with maximum payoffs so that your time is well spent.

Uses of Pareto Charts

The Pareto chart can be used for continuous improvement in the following ways:

- You can use it to focus your attention on the "vital few" instead of the "trivial many" problems or processes needing attention in a way that has visual impact.
- You can use it to decide which problem to pursue.
- You can use it to identify the more influential causes of your problem.
- You can use it to show changes in performance over time. For example, if you achieve an improvement as a result of tackling one of the important root causes, that cause should drop in severity, losing its place as the front-runner on your Pareto chart.

Following are some illustrations of such uses:

- *Use in selecting an improvement opportunity.* The Pareto chart in figure 10-23 was based on patient survey results and was used to help a nursing team determine which three problems to work on. "Listening" to the chart, the team decided to work on (1) communicating more effectively about what the patient can expect, (2) answering calls more rapidly, and (3) improving friendliness.
- *Use in identifying a powerful cause.* The Pareto chart shown in figure 10-24 (p. 131) was used by an improvement team to compare the relative length of delays at each step in the process for patients entering the hospital through the emergency room, from the moment an inpatient admissions decision was made to the time the patient arrived at a critical care bed. This chart suggested that waiting for both the physician and

Figure 10-22. Example of a Pareto Chart

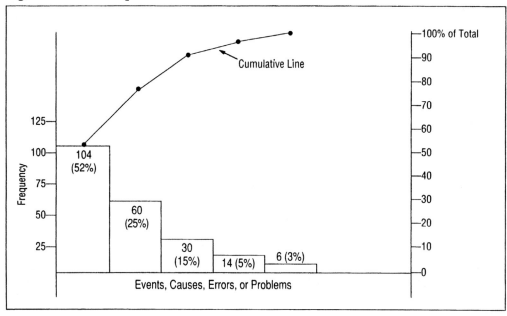

Figure 10-23. Pareto Chart Used to Determine Which Problems to Target for Improvement

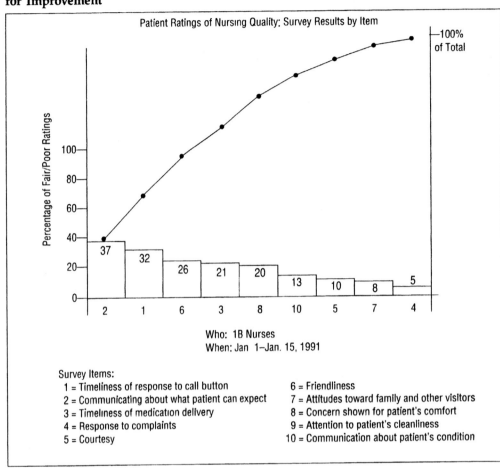

Patient Ratings of Nursing Quality: Survey Results by Item

Who: 1B Nurses
When: Jan 1–Jan. 15, 1991

Survey Items:
1 = Timeliness of response to call button
2 = Communicating about what patient can expect
3 = Timeliness of medication delivery
4 = Response to complaints
5 = Courtesy
6 = Friendliness
7 = Attitudes toward family and other visitors
8 = Concern shown for patient's comfort
9 = Attention to patient's cleanliness
10 = Communication about patient's condition

the environment to be prepared were the two steps in the process that consumed the most unnecessary time. If these causes of delays could be alleviated, the overall delay would be significantly reduced.

How to Construct a Pareto Chart

The following eight steps should be followed to derive useful data from a Pareto chart:

1. Determine a time period for data collection and design a check sheet for gathering data during that time period.
2. Collect the data and record them on the check sheet.
3. Summarize your data on a Pareto work sheet, rearranging your categories from the check sheet in descending order of scores.
4. Based on your data, make a Pareto chart that shows your results in descending order from left to right, with the largest category on the left, followed by the next-largest category, and so on. The vertical axis on the left should represent the count, or frequency. Categories, problem types, or causes should be along the horizontal axis.
5. On the right axis, indicate percentage of total.
6. Add each bar to the sum of the bar(s) to its immediate left. Calculate the percentage of total above each bar and place the percentage on the graph in its

Figure 10-24. Pareto Chart (without Cumulative Line) Showing Delay from Admission to Arrival in Unit

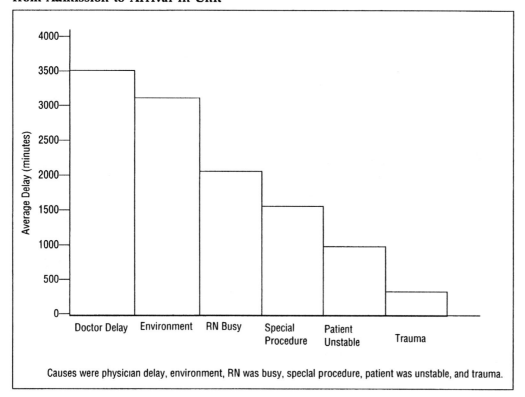

Causes were physician delay, environment, RN was busy, special procedure, patient was unstable, and trauma.

Reprinted, with permission, from Holston Valley Hospital and Medical Center, Kingsport, TN, 1990.

relationship to the percentage of total indicated on the scale to the right of the graph.

7. Indicate the title of the graph and how the data were calculated for future reference.
8. Redraw the chart over time so that you can see changes.

Case Example

A patient representative is tracking complaints and wants to determine the most frequently recurring ones because these contribute to patient dissatisfaction more often than those voiced less frequently. She plans to initiate prevention efforts designed to address these vital few.

First, she develops a check sheet to record, over a 15-week period, instances of complaints in eight categories (see figure 10-25). She then summarizes the check sheet data on a Pareto work sheet, rearranging the complaint types in order of decreasing frequency and calculating cumulative frequency (figure 10-26, p. 133). The results are then depicted on a Pareto chart that shows that discourteous staff and problems with patients' rooms and physical surroundings are the most frequent reasons for complaining (figure 10-27, p. 134). In fact, if those problems were addressed successfully, as much as 60 percent of the total number of complaints could be eliminated.

After a year of well-conceived actions designed to reduce the frequency of complaints about staff discourtesy and physical plant problems, the patient representative drew a before-and-after Pareto chart to see the results (figure 10-28, p. 135). She felt that complaints about staff discourtesy and physical plant problems should decline in frequency compared to other complaint types for which no remedies had been attempted. She was also interested in whether the *total* number of complaints, not just the relative proportion

Figure 10-25. Check Sheet of Patient Complaints Postdischarge

								Summary of Raw Data, Month of January								
Complaint Type	1	2	3	4	5	6	7	8	9	10	11	12	13	14	15	15-Day Total
Problem with room/physical plant	6	2	5	8	6	6	4	8	7	6	4	9	2	2	8	83
Discourteous staff	10	6	6	9	12	9	8	10	16	14	10	8	4	6	8	142
Complaints about doctor	2	4	8	4	2	1	1	2	4	9	6	2	3	1	1	50
Lack of attention to specific personal needs	2	2	4	2	1	1	2	4	6	2	2	4	6	2	3	43
Dissatisfaction with length of stay	1	4	2	3	1	1	2	1	1	2	2	1	1	2	2	26
Poor TV programs	1	0	0	2	1	0	0	0	0	2	0	0	0	1	0	7
Visitor policy problems	2	4	2	2	0	1	1	1	2	1	1	1	0	0	1	19
Staff incompetence	2	1	0	0	0	0	0	0	2	2	0	0	1	0	0	8

Total Complaints: 378

Figure 10-26. Pareto Work Sheet of Patient Complaints Postdischarge

Complaint Type	Number of Complaints	Percentage of Total	Cumulative Percentage
Discourteous staff	142	37.6	37.6
Problems with room, physical plant	83	22.0	59.6
Complaints about doctor	50	13.2	72.8
Lack of attention to specific personal needs	43	11.4	84.2
Dissatisfaction with length of stay	26	6.9	91.1
Visitor policy problems	19	5.0	96.1
Other (lump several low-scoring complaint categories)	15	3.9	100.0

of complaints, had been reduced. Therefore, she depicted the total number of complaints on a stacked bar chart, which showed the decline in the number of complaining customers that occurred as a result of action to reduce just the two most frequently recurring complaint types (figure 10-29, p. 136). She found that the total number of complaints dropped from 330 to 270, or 18 percent, a reduction largely attributable to fewer complaints related to what were formerly the top two causes.

Precautions

Note the following precautions in the use of Pareto charts:

- The Pareto chart assumes that quantity equals importance, which is certainly not always the case. For example, one complaint about malpractice is more important than 10 complaints about dingy paint in patients' rooms. When you are measuring errors, some that may occur less frequently may have far more serious consequences than others. You need to use common sense when you interpret your Pareto chart.
- The Pareto chart merely gives you a visual picture of the frequency of various problems, events, or causes. To make decisions based on the results, you might want to apply criteria other than frequency. For example, cause number 1 on your chart might be more difficult to address than cause number 2. Or a solution to cause number 3 might be short-term and easy and cost nothing. So, why not begin with cause number 3 and experience an easy success? You do not have to make the Pareto chart winners your priorities. You need to consider the results and discuss them (perhaps using a decision matrix) in view of other criteria for selecting a problem or cause.

Figure 10-27. Pareto Chart of Patient Complaints Postdischarge

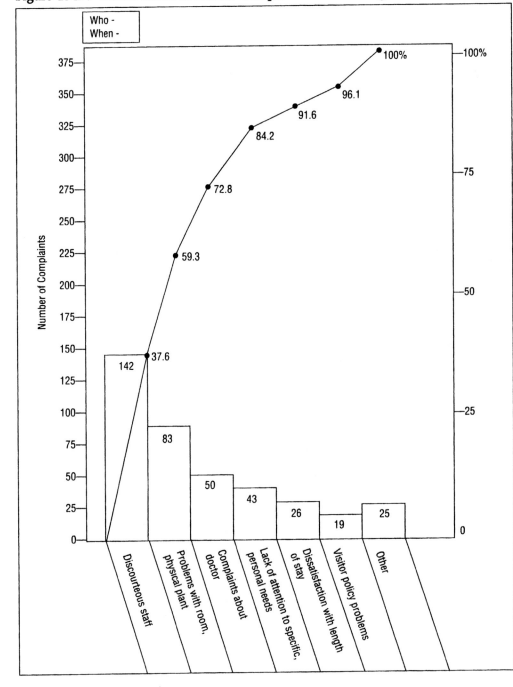

Figure 10-28. Before-and-after Pareto Chart

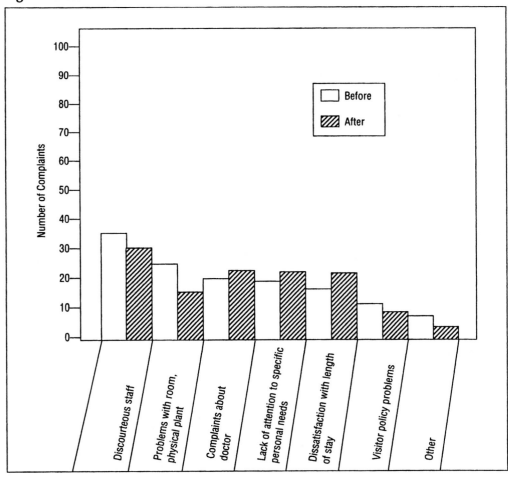

Figure 10-29. Stacked Bar Chart

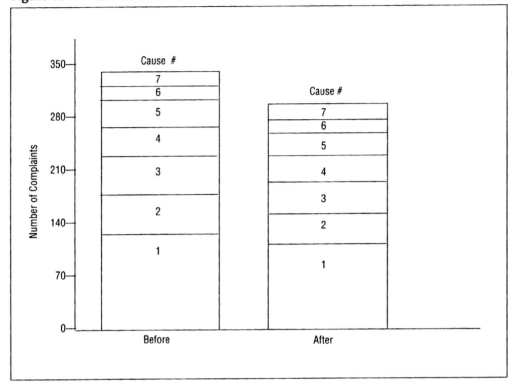

☐ Tool 7: Trend Charts, Run Charts, and Control Charts

Trend charts, run charts, and *control charts* are visual displays of performance over time.

Trend Charts

Trend charts are performance plotters that can be used to monitor the movement in your long-range average and thus draw conclusions about whether performance is moving up, moving down, or staying the same. Figure 10-30 shows a basic trend chart. As shown, the measured value is on the *y* axis (the percentage of patients seen within 30 minutes) and the time scale (days) is on the *x* axis. Each day, the percentage of patients seen within 30 minutes is reflected by placing a data point at the intersection of the date and the appropriate percentage. Then, by connecting the data points, you can see trends as the percentage dips and swings. Shifts in the average level of performance can thus be monitored. In tracking the performance of most processes, you can expect fluctuations. When you see a noticeable pattern of dips and swings emerging, you will know that something has triggered a change. This should signal you to investigate further to understand what happened and to do what is needed, for example, to hold onto gains (in the case of improvements) or to identify and solve the problem in the case of drops in performance. With a trend chart, you need to watch performance over several time periods to notice trends rather than single fluctuations.

How to Construct a Trend Chart
The following steps should be followed in constructing a trend chart:

1. Determine what you want to measure. You might measure customer satisfaction scores on a survey question, number of people served, percentage of on-time

Figure 10-30. Basic Trend Chart

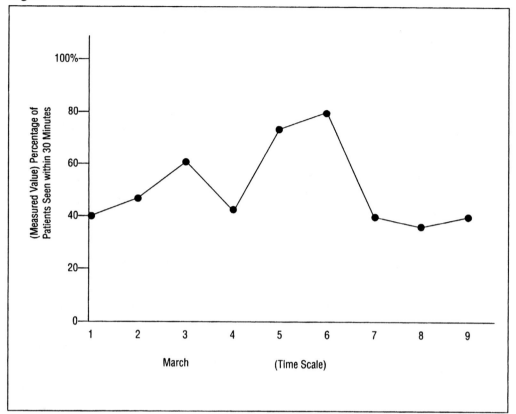

deliveries of medications per day, X ray retakes, errors, productivity, complaints, on-time delivery of service, and so forth. Label what you are measuring clearly along the *y* (vertical) axis of your chart.

2. Determine your measurement schedule, that is, the time intervals you want to include on the *x* (horizontal) axis of your trend chart. You can use months, quarters, weeks, mornings, hours, and so on. Mark these clearly along the *x* axis of your chart.

3. Collect measurements according to your schedule by recording each data point on a run chart or control chart (see the next two sections for further explanation of these charts). To create a separate trend chart that summarizes your results for a time period (for example, a month or quarter), average all your measurements for the time period on your run or control chart and reflect that average with one point on your trend chart.

4. Connect your data points so that you can see the trends more vividly.

Uses of Trend Charts
Trend charts can be used in the following ways:

- To address the question, "How are we doing?"
- To help monitor and summarize performance and changes in performance over time. Trend charts are great as progress plotters when you are taking steps to make improvements and want to see whether your experiments are paying off.
- To serve as powerful communication devices. Trend charts can be used to raise staff awareness of performance, either triggering pride and celebration in response to improvement or mobilizing toward improvement in response to declines in

performance. Some department heads paper a busy hallway wall with a collection of trend charts that show performance related to the department's key customer requirements. People naturally feel good when they see the performance lines creeping upward. And they became concerned when the performance lines dip downward. When you make trend charts visible, they become powerful tools for engaging staff energy and concern in your continuous improvement efforts.

Following are two examples of trend chart uses. In the first, an important team was tracking physician satisfaction with the hospital. As team members pursued improvements, they instituted two experiments to see whether they could heighten satisfaction. The first measure taken was to offer a physician referral service to help affiliated physicians increase patient volume. The second measure was to offer practice enhancement workshops to physicians and their office staff. The trend chart in figure 10-31 shows the timing of each experimental improvement and the resulting rise in physician satisfaction that followed each, leveling off over the past few months at around 70 percent.

In the second example, an outpatient clinic was determined to see every scheduled patient within 20 minutes of his or her appointment time. The trend chart in figure 10-32 shows the actual percentage of patients seen daily within the 20-minute time frame compared to the clinic's target of 90 percent.

Tips
Following are some pointers to help you interpret trend charts more accurately:

- Avoid drawing conclusions from a single point on your trend chart. Look at the whole or changing picture. For instance, a single downward fluctuation in your average might not be important. But if you saw your average slipping over time, you would know that you have a downward trend that needs attention and not just a single aberration.
- Record countermeasures or improvements on your graph so that you can see performance levels before and after the change.

Figure 10-31. Trend Chart Showing Physician Satisfaction after Two Experimental Improvements

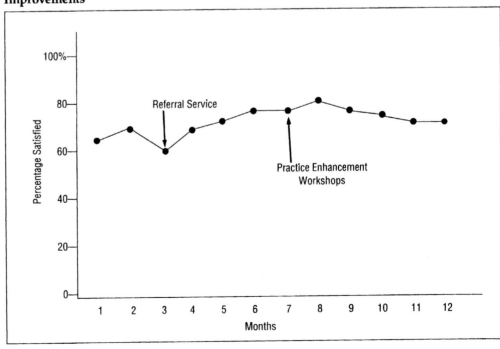

Figure 10-32. Trend Chart Showing Percentage of Patients Seen within 30 Minutes

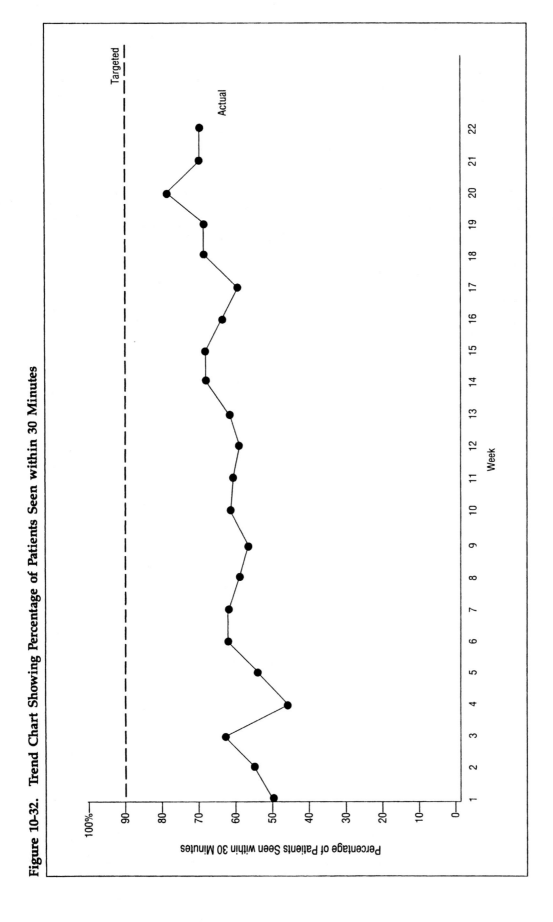

Run Charts

Variation is natural to every process. Fluctuations that fall within calculated limits are said to result from common causes or variations built into the process. You can only make improvements by changing your process, because these fluctuations are built into it and are normal. But when measurement points fall outside these limits, there is a special cause that calls for investigation because it is not expected from that process.

Both run charts and control charts help you to track performance, determine whether performance is in control, and identify special causes of variation that must be understood and changed to get the process back in control.

The run chart differs from the trend chart in that it tracks *individual data points* and not the average for a time period. Run charts are simply easy-to-construct plots of data recorded in time sequence. By analyzing the patterns shown in run charts, you should gain valuable clues about whether the variation has special or common causes. When you see no symptoms of special causes, you can project the long-term performance of the process. When you do see symptoms of special causes, the process is out of control and you need to investigate those special causes of variation.

How to Construct a Run Chart
The following steps should be undertaken in developing a run chart:

1. Construct a chart with the vertical or *y* axis representing your variable and the horizontal or *x* axis representing the time sequence.
2. Plot each data point in time sequence and draw a line connecting the points to form a line chart.
3. Find the median of the data. The median is the value that divides your data into two equal parts; half of your data points are above it, and half are below it. To find the median, count the number of data points you've recorded on your chart. Then, holding a ruler horizontally, move it from the top of the chart downward until half of your data points are either showing or along the ruler's edge. Draw a line along the ruler's edge across your chart and label this line the median, or *x*.

How to Interpret a Run Chart
A *run* is a connected sequence of points on the same side of your median line. You analyze the run chart by interpreting these runs. Different run patterns suggest special causes of variation that warrant investigation (see figure 10-33):

- *Run length.* Count the number of consecutive data points on one side of the median. A run of seven data points or more is considered abnormal and suggests special causes.
- *Freaks.* Dramatic aberrations, or *freaks*, suggest a process out of control.
- *Trends.* A run of seven or more points in a continuous upward or downward direction also is considered abnormal.
- *Sudden shifts.* A sudden shift in a different direction needs looking into.
- *Cycling.* A zigzag pattern of up-and-down movements is also abnormal and suggests special causes.

Look at the patterns in your run chart and ask: "What questions does the pattern raise? What special causes do we need to investigate?"

Control Charts

Control charts are run charts with one more level of sophistication and helpfulness. They show statistically determined limits drawn on both sides of the line indicating deviations

Figure 10-33. Run Charts with Different Distributions

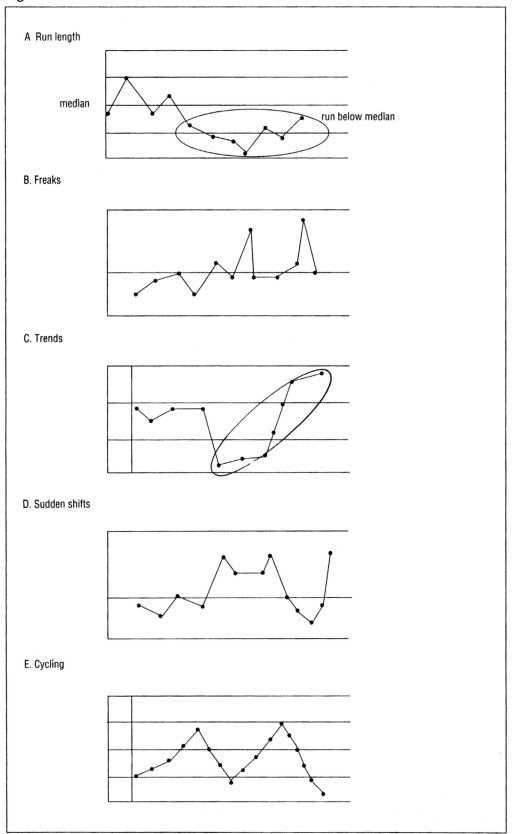

from the average. They tell you whether variations in performance around your average are within normal limits (due to *common* causes) or are out of control (due to *special* causes). You use control charts to see whether your current process is consistently producing predictable degrees of fluctuation (see figure 10-34).

Control charts require the use of simple statistical techniques. Numerous computer software programs can do the charting and the statistics for you once you enter your data points. Once you become accustomed to using the simpler technique of the run chart, which requires no statistics, the appropriate next step would be to learn to use control charts. (For a complete explanation, see Pyzdek's *Pyzdek's Guide to SPC*,[2] Goal/QPC's *Memory Jogger*,[3] and Ozeki's *Handbook of Quality Tools*.[4])

Figure 10-34. Control Chart

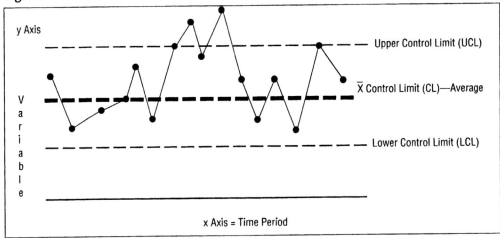

Precautions about Trend, Run, and Control Charts

Note the following precautions in the use of trend charts, run charts, and control charts:

- If you make changes in the process during the data-collection period, your data become misleading. Be careful how you interpret them in that circumstance.
- Just because a process appears to be under control does not mean that it is meeting customer expectations. It just means that you are getting "consistent" performance, that is, performance that stays predictably close to your average level for that process. Imagine a short-staffed or inefficient admissions function in a hospital. It may be that incoming patients predictably wait approximately three hours to be admitted. There are fluctuations around that three-hour mark, but they fall within statistically defined limits indicating the consistency of this waiting time. However, that doesn't mean that patients are satisfied with that long wait. The information tells you that your current process can be expected to produce three-hour waits and that, to reduce waiting time, you have to change the process. Processes that are in control are still important focal points for continuous improvement if (1) they fail to meet customer expectations or (2) they create other problems for the organization, such as costing too much, consuming too much staff time, or causing staff frustration.

References

1. *Instructor's Guide*. Wilton, CT: Juran Institute, 1989, p. 2.

2. Pyzdek, T. *Pyzdek's Guide to SPC*. Tucson: Quality American, Inc., and ASQC Quality Press, 1989.

3. Goal/QPC. *Memory Jogger*. Methuen, MA: Goal/QPC, 1988.

4. Ozeki, K., and Asaka, T. *Handbook of Quality Tools*. Cambridge, MA: Productivity Press, 1990.

Chapter 11
Tools for Targeting Improvements

The use of visual tools to solve problems and make improvements facilitates the process of reaching consensus, making quality decisions, and building confidence in those decisions. Like any tools, those presented here are meant to extend your power and flexibility. Sometimes, straightforward discussion will be all you need to build consensus and make decisions that are appropriate and efficient. Other times, the tools we describe here will be invaluable for moving forward through the stages of process improvement, organizing a variety of thoughts and ideas, visualizing relationships that are otherwise difficult to see, speeding up consensus building, or unlocking a stymied group.

There are no prescriptions or fail-proof sequences for applying tools to problems. The challenge is to equip yourself with a diversity of tools and be willing to experiment. As you approach a process improvement, ask yourself, "What could help us here?" Then, pull that tool from your tool kit and try it. If it helps, great; if it does not help, try something else. With experience, your batting average for applying tools appropriately and reaping their benefits will improve dramatically. The following tools for solving problems and making improvements are described in this chapter:

- Flowcharts
- Brainstorming
- Affinity charts
- Relationship diagrams
- Cause-and-effect diagrams
- Force-field analysis
- Decision matrices
- Tree diagrams
- Action planning

☐ Tool 8: Flowcharts

The easiest way to get a grip on a process is to draw a picture of it. Simply put, that is what a *flowchart* is—a picture of a process. Like a road map, a flowchart vividly portrays, sequentially and in picture form, every activity or step in a process intended to lead to an output. Typically, no one individual in a group knows the entire process. By mapping out the process, group members can gain a shared understanding of it and use their shared understanding to collect data, narrow down the problem, focus discussion of the process, and identify resources. Although it seems obvious that to improve and control a process you must first understand it, many managers and teams try to attack problems and make improvements without taking the critical first step of creating a flowchart.

Flowcharts range from the simple to the complex. A simple flowchart is a crude picture of process steps in sequence, each contained in a box and connected with arrows to the steps that come before and after (see figure 11-1). Even a simple flowchart can be extremely powerful when you want to understand your current situation, pinpoint opportunities for improvement, revamp your process to reflect the improvements, and build the changes into standard operating procedure. A more enlightening flowchart, and the kind that is more helpful in group problem solving, includes symbols for activities, decisions, waits, stops-and-starts, arrows, and documentation (see figure 11-2). With these more precise symbols, the group can specify the exact nature of an element in the process, whether it is an activity, a decision, or a wait. For example, when you reach the analysis stage, you can look at all the wait symbols and ask whether and why they are necessary. Or you can look at the decision points and clarify the criteria for making the right decisions.

How to Construct a Flowchart

The following steps should facilitate the construction of a flowchart:

1. List the steps involved in a process using direct observation, brainstorming, or consultation with the people responsible for each step. It helps to be thorough when you ask questions about inputs, throughputs, and outputs of the process overall and at each step. For example:
   • Questions about inputs:
     −Who provides the input (information, a chart, the patient, an order, a result)?
     −Who receives the input (which position/department)?
   • Questions about throughput:
     −What is the first thing done with that input? And then what?
     −What checks or tests are performed at each step?
     −What happens if the step does not pass the test?
   • Questions about outputs:
     −Who receives the output? Where does the product or service produced by this process go?
     −What do they do with it? And then what?
2. Arrange the activities and decisions in chronological order, depicting each with the appropriate symbol. You know when you're finished if:
   • You've connected all inputs to outputs.
   • The flowchart shows both the parallel activities and the sequence of events.

Figure 11-1. Simple Flowchart

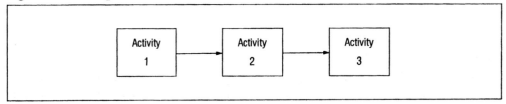

Figure 11-2. Flowchart Symbols

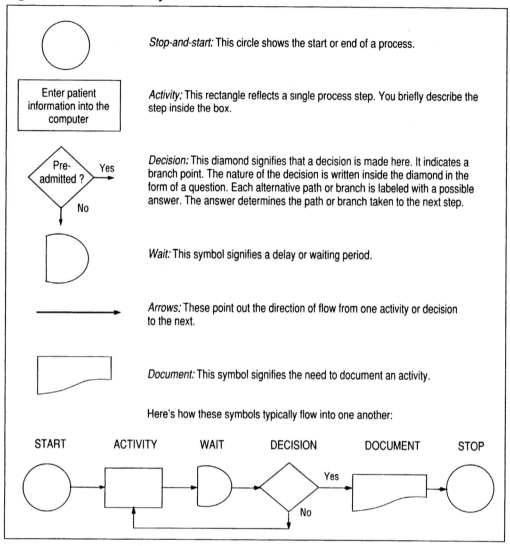

- The chart includes all decisions that affect the flow of the process.
- The chart shows all possible paths that things, work, and/or people take, even when unexpected events occur or rework must be done.
- The chart reflects reality, not fiction or intention.

3. If different people or departments are responsible for different steps in the process (as is so often true in health care organizations), list the responsible parties across the top of your chart. Then, without losing chronological sequence, place each activity and decision in the process under the people or department responsible for it.

4. If possible, do a walk-through or observation of the actual process to verify the process as drawn.

Tips

Following are a few pointers that can help expedite the process of flowcharting:

- Make sure you involve the right people in making the flowchart, including those who actually do the work, suppliers to the process, customers of the process, and managers or supervisors involved in its control. It also helps to have a facilitator who can help people through the flowchart design process itself.

- Because many processes have many steps, use many sheets of flip chart paper, Post-it™ notes, or Sticky Wall™ sprayed on flip chart paper so that you can move steps around flexibly until you think you have positioned all of them correctly.
- When you are investigating a complicated process, it helps first to do a crude flowchart that includes only the major steps and then to break all the major steps down into substeps.
- It may take a substantial amount of time to make a flowchart, often more than one sitting. Remind yourself that it is worth the effort because your data collection and problem solving rely on your flowchart's accuracy and thoroughness.

Examples of Flowcharts

Following are various flowcharts used for somewhat different purposes.

Flowchart of Physicians' Orders for Medication
The flowchart in figure 11-3 shows the process from the time a physician writes a medication order to the time the order is filled. It shows three critical points at which rework is often necessary: (1) when the physicians' orders are illegible, (2) when the nurse cannot understand the order, and (3) when either the pharmacy needs clarification of the order or the medication is not in the hospital's formulary. By identifying these points, an improvement team can see ways to reduce costly, time-consuming instances of rework.

In this case, the flowchart was helpful in developing justification for physician order entry into the hospital's patient care computer system. If the physician were to enter the medication order directly, two steps in the process would be eliminated: (1) The unit secretary would not have to check for legibility and call the physician when orders were illegible, and (2) the pharmacist would not have to check the availability of the medication on the hospital's formulary and call the physician in the event of a problem.

Flowchart of Admission from Emergency Department to a Medical–Surgical Bed
The Quality First team at Holston Valley Hospital and Medical Center, in Kingsport, Tennessee, used a SIPOC chart to help them develop their flowchart of the process from admission from the emergency department (E.D.) to a surgical bed (see figure 11-4). Use

Figure 11-3. Flowchart of Physician's Order for Medication

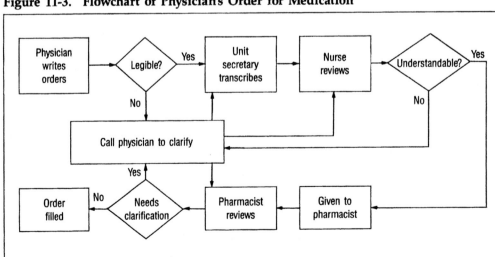

Reprinted, with permission, from St. Clair Hospital, Pittsburgh, 1990.

Figure 11-4. SIPOC Chart of Admissions Process from Emergency Department to a Surgical Bed

Suppliers	Inputs	Processes	Outputs	Customer
Physician	Sick patient	Order to be admitted	Order written	Nurse
Nurse	Written order	Notified admitting	Notify patient	Admitting
Admitting	Notified of bed	Patient gets bed	Bed	E.D. nurse
E.D. nurse	Notifies floor nurse	Completes order	Completed order	Floor nurse
Floor nurse	Transferred patient	Receives patient	Patient on floor	Patient

Reprinted, with permission, from Holston Valley Hospital and Medical Center, Kingsport, TN, 1990.

of this chart provided an organized way for team members to identify their suppliers (S), inputs (I), processes (P), outputs (O), and customers (C). Once the SIPOC chart was complete, it was easier to draw the flowchart, which is shown in figure 11-5. This "matrix" flowchart shows all the steps involving the patient and all the responsibilities within the domains of patient registration, the E.D. nurse, the E.D. secretary, the physician, and the floor nurse.

The team used this flowchart to pursue ways to reduce delays from the time a decision is made to admit an E.D. patient to the time the patient is received with a room assignment on a medical–surgical floor. By mapping the process up front, the team could collect data on the length of time consumed at each step in the process and then focus in on the process activities that most contributed to unnecessary delays.

Service Blueprint of Health Screening Service

Service blueprinting is a variation of flowcharting. You draw a simple flowchart, or blueprint, of the customer's pathway through the service and ask, "At which points along this pathway do we have problems, rework, wasted energy, staff or customer frustration, or other quality problems?"

Following is an example of how a small health screening service benefited from using service blueprints. The screening service, which targets senior citizens, was having problems with cramped quarters and excessive dependency on other hospital services. The improvement team developed a service blueprint that mapped out the customer's pathway from promotion to completion of his or her tests (see figure 11-6, p. 149). By mapping out each step along the patient's pathway through the service, the interdependencies among departments and the points at which service failed became evident. The screening service then set out to streamline the blueprint and from the revised blueprint (see figure 11-7, p. 150) was able to streamline operations and strengthen weaknesses. The service eliminated three of its interdepartmental dependencies and reduced the number of different offices patients had to visit for evaluation and testing by conducting on-site tests. And by converting nurses' offices into health screening areas, the service was able to solve the problem of tight physical facilities.

In this example, the use of blueprinting facilitated an understanding of the customer's view of the service; helped focus the collection of feedback from staff, patients, and physicians; and helped the people involved in the service to see and track interdepartmental interactions, isolate and identify fail points, design an enhanced service, define needed resources, pinpoint step-by-step the costs involved, and ultimately better define performance expectations for every step along the patient's pathway.

Uses of Flowcharts

Flowcharts are the cornerstone of logical approaches to both quality control and process improvement. They can be used in any of the following ways:

Figure 11-5. Flowchart of Admission from Emergency Department to Surgical Bed

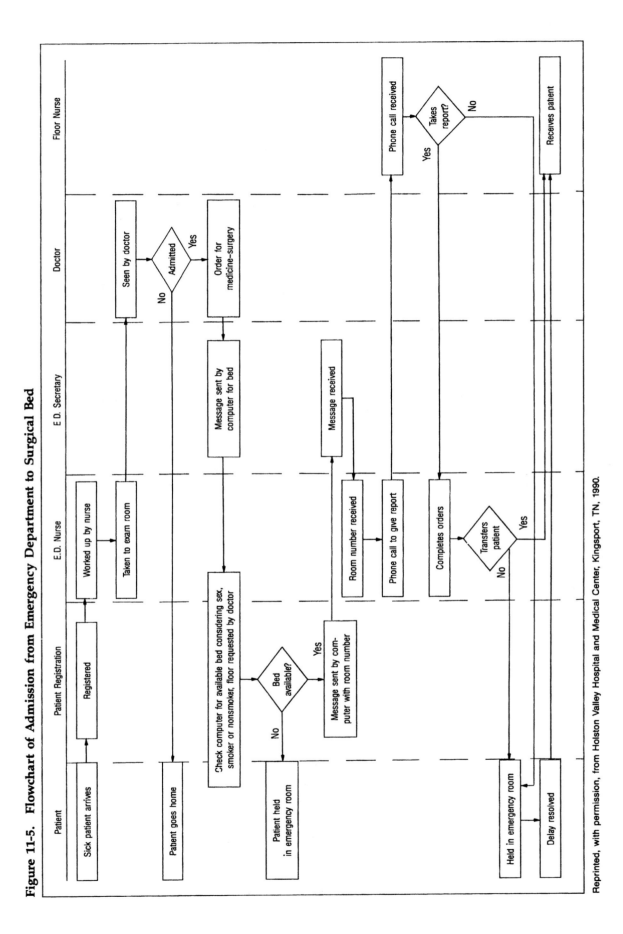

Reprinted, with permission, from Holston Valley Hospital and Medical Center, Kingsport, TN, 1990.

Figure 11-6. Service Blueprint of Health Screening Service

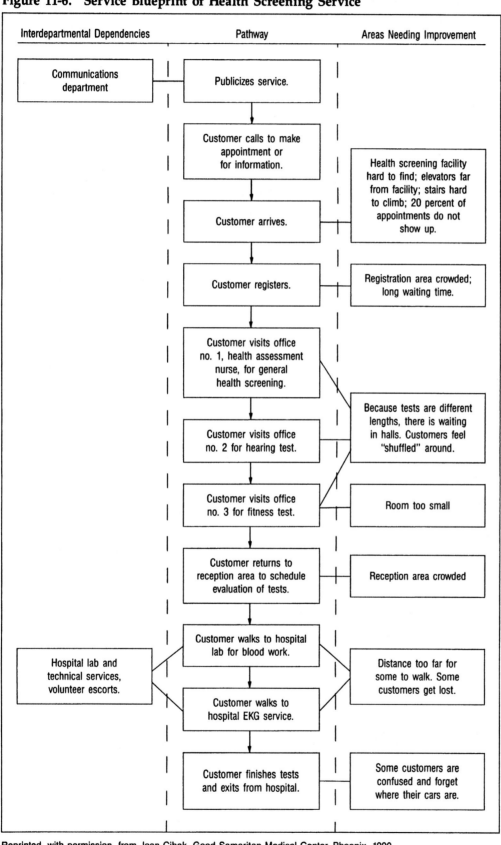

Reprinted, with permission, from Joan Cihak, Good Samaritan Medical Center, Phoenix, 1990.

Figure 11-7. Revised Service Blueprint of Health Screening Service

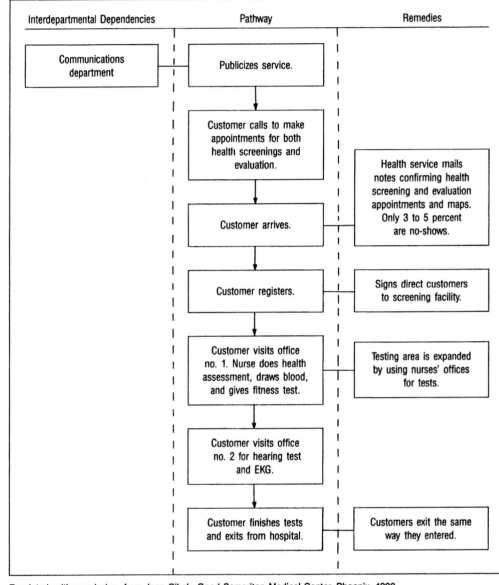

Reprinted, with permission, from Joan Cihak, Good Samaritan Medical Center, Phoenix, 1990.

- Flowcharts help you and your group to crystallize the way the process works *now*. To design process improvements, you need to begin by clearly portraying the process you already follow to see its logic or lack of logic.
- A group or team can use a flowchart to understand and walk through even a complex process without having to leave the conference room. Throughout a problem-solving process, flowcharts can provide the anchor and point of reference needed to keep the focus clear.
- After mapping out the current process, it is much easier to figure out what kind of information is needed to move forward. By methodically collecting information about every step, you can identify bottlenecks or missteps and the extent to which they affect your results. When you define problems in this way, you gain confidence that you are focusing on the right problems and improvement opportunities.
- Flowcharts help you to identify problems. You can examine a flowchart of current reality and, after collecting data about each step, identify bottlenecks. Or you can

draw a "real" and "ideal" flowchart, identifying discrepancies that reveal problems. For each process step, you can ask:
—Is this activity necessary or redundant?
—What value does this activity add to the process?
—What is the cost of this activity?
—How do we prevent errors, problems, or variation in this activity?
—Is there a way we can check for problems or errors in this activity?
—How well does our check detect problems?

- Flowcharts help groups or teams to make conscious decisions about the scope or focus of their improvement effort, deciding which step or steps they want to modify and thus preventing the discussion from meandering in a time-consuming and disorganized fashion.
- People who help you to create the flowchart become engaged in quality improvement and continue to suggest improvements long after the flowchart design process has ended.
- A new flowchart of the revised process after improvements have been made can help you to clarify the process, expectations, and roles, as well as train the people involved. When people engaged in a process can visualize it clearly, they can control it instead of feeling controlled by it. Also, when employees see how they fit into a process, they can more clearly visualize their suppliers and customers, a powerful aid to better communication across departmental lines and between work groups.
- After doing a trial run of your improved process and making the necessary adjustments, you can graphically show in a refined flowchart the new process that is to become the standard operating procedure until further notice.

☐ Tool 9: Brainstorming

Brainstorming is a quick, powerful, and energizing technique to elicit from a group (an improvement team, a work group, a customer group, or a focus group) an outpouring or list of ideas, perceptions, problems, opportunities, questions, possible causes, dimensions of a problem, alternate solutions, and so forth. It is an extremely versatile tool. In fact, it is often used as one part of many other process improvement methods.

Specifically, brainstorming helps a group to generate many thoughts or ideas in a very short time, without judgment or discussion along the way. The key to its power is the phrase *without judgment or discussion*. In a typical group discussion, someone expresses a thought and others comment on it, question it, or judge it either positively or negatively. The result is that people focus in on that one idea before all other possible ideas have a chance to emerge. Group members might spend their precious time talking about one thought when the time would be better spent generating a whole list of thoughts and then homing in on those they believe are worthy of more time and attention.

Also, in typical group discussions, when people respond to one another's ideas with judgments, others are discouraged from speaking up for fear of having their thoughts questioned or attacked or, in the case of positive responses, for fear of saying something and *not* getting the kind of compliment or acknowledgment received by others. This also slows down the flow of ideas.

Brainstorming, on the other hand, encourages the flow and fluency of people's thoughts. Because judgments are taboo, creativity is sparked and people loosen up as they have nothing to fear from others' responses.

How to Conduct Brainstorming

Brainstorming has three phases: generation, clarification, and evaluation.

151

Chapter 11

The Generation Phase

The leader reviews the rules of brainstorming with group members, clearly states the question or purpose, writes it as the header on a flip chart, and then invites and records responses. This phase can be either structured or unstructured. When you use the structured approach, each person must offer a thought or idea in turn or pass until the next round. This encourages quiet or shy people to speak up but may also cause people to feel uncomfortable pressure. When you use the unstructured or free-for-all approach, group members speak up whenever they have a thought, in no particular order. This method tends to create a more relaxed mood but runs the risk that outspoken or particularly enthusiastic people might dominate the session.

In either approach, the rules are the same:

- Quantity, not quality. The more, the merrier.
- Discussion, judgment, and criticism are all suspended during the generation process.
- It's fine to piggyback or build on others' ideas.
- Practicality is unimportant; far-out ideas are welcome.
- Three-word minimum per idea; otherwise, it's difficult for people to know what is really being suggested.
- Six- or seven-word maximum; otherwise, you'll hear speeches.

Following are some tips that may facilitate the process:

- Record *every* idea in the speaker's own words for all to see. Use a flip chart to record the ideas.
- Do not let people break the rules. Use a whimsical signal such as a bicycle horn or a red flag to signal a violation. This enables you to avoid a verbal reprimand when someone has judged, criticized, or otherwise broken the rules. The signal is especially helpful if the group is just learning how to brainstorm.
- Brainstorming should move quickly. Give people a 15-second warning before ending it so that they can spill out any ideas left unsaid. A typical brainstorming session lasts between 5 and 10 minutes.

The Clarification Phase

After the list is generated, the group reviews it to ensure that everyone is clear about what all the items mean. Because the generation phase has a "quantity, not quality" emphasis, some items are expressed in vague terms. At this stage, people are encouraged to ask, "What was meant by this?" This clarification is important before ideas are judged so that in later discussion unclear ideas are not dismissed along with unworkable ideas.

The Evaluation Phase

The group considers the list and rules out duplications, irrelevant ideas, or ideas considered beyond its scope or power. Affinity charting (the next tool discussed in this chapter) is a great technique for seeing patterns within an array of brainstormed ideas. A decision matrix would then be helpful in evaluating the ideas according to such criteria as potential impact on problem, costliness, ease or speed of implementation, and so forth. In other words, screen and sort to narrow down the list of ideas to a select few.

Uses of Brainstorming

Obviously, the list of possibilities for using brainstorming is infinite. Here's a partial list:

- Brainstorm problems your group might want to tackle.
- Brainstorm alternative solutions to a problem.

152

- Brainstorm factors that contribute to a problem in your hunt for root causes. For instance, brainstorm the possible causes on a cause-and-effect diagram (tool 12 in this chapter).
- Use brainstorming to generate alternative problem statements before targeting one.
- Brainstorm "driving forces" and "restraining forces" in a force-field analysis (tool 13 in this chapter).
- Brainstorm elements to be clustered in an affinity chart.
- Brainstorm the branches in a tree diagram (tool 15 in this chapter).
- Brainstorm obstacles that might interfere with successful implementation of a plan you have developed.
- Brainstorm the individual elements of a process before organizing and sequencing them in a flowchart.
- Brainstorm benefits of an innovation in preparation for "selling" it to your boss.
- Brainstorm questions you might use to survey customer satisfaction.
- Brainstorm information that might shed light on the essence or causes of a problem.
- Brainstorm components of an action plan before you sequence the steps and assign responsibility.

Following are two examples of the use of brainstorming. In the first example, the manager of the dietary department worked with staff to brainstorm a list of ways the department could better satisfy the hospital's employees regarding food services. The brainstorming session generated the following ideas:

- Add a cashier to speed up checkout.
- Offer a low-fat, sugar-free option.
- Replace wobbly chairs.
- Have line workers say hello.
- Break the routine by offering ethnic meals.
- Offer monthly meal ticket for a fair price.
- Expand hours for day and evening people.
- Open for two hours at night.
- Add healthy options to vending machines.
- Sell goodies in take-home, microwavable packages.
- Post calorie and fat content on entrees.
- Expand the no-smoking area.
- Play music.
- Have guerilla theater or five-minute concerts by employees in the cafeteria.
- Invite feedback on the quality of the entrees.
- Survey employees about likes and dislikes.
- Do periodic focus groups with employees to get new ideas.

Afterward, the group used a decision matrix (tool 14) to rate these ideas according to their likely impact on employee satisfaction, their cost, and the difficulty of implementing them. They then selected two ideas to pursue further.

In the second example, a liaison team, consisting of people from nursing and environmental services, brainstormed possible causes of problems affecting their service partnership. Their brainstorming generated the following causes:

- It's not clear whom to call with problems.
- There's no feedback about when problems will be resolved.
- The pecking order creates barriers to getting needs addressed fast.
- Nurses think they are more important because they take care of patients.
- Housekeepers feel unvalued by some nurse managers.
- The environmental supervisor is rarely available.

- There's no clear system for getting a problem taken care of.
- Nursing does not give environmental services enough notice once a room is vacated.

The team voted to select the two causes of communication problems with the most powerful impact and then explored ways to resolve them.

☐ Tool 10: Affinity Charts

Affinity charting is a process for generating an abundance of ideas, opinions, perceptions, issues, or activities and then organizing them into natural clusters of related items (figure 11-8). The resulting clusters are easier to discuss, manage, and manipulate than the large number of individual elements generated originally. Also, patterns begin to emerge that help make sense of many different ideas.

Figure 11-8. From Brainstorm to Affinity Chart

A. Initial Brainstorm

Solutions to problems
Results that will satisfy administrators
Good feelings among us
Happier patients
Fewer fires to put out
Harmony among us
Faith in possibility of solving problems
Teamwork among us
Teamwork between departments; less turf
More physician cooperation
Happier physicians
No more cynicism
Better relationships between departments
Less frustration when things go wrong
More efficient operations
Better problem-solving skills among us

B. Resulting Two-Part Affinity Chart

Our Team's Objectives

Concrete Improvements	*Heightened Customer Satisfaction*
Solutions to problems	Happier patients
Fewer fires to put out	More physician cooperation
Results that satisfy administrators	Happier physicians

The Values We Want to Guide Us

Better Interdepartmental Collaboration	*Growth/Gratification for Team Members*
Better relationships between departments	Better problem-solving skills among us
Less frustration when things go wrong	Faith in prospect of solving problems
More efficient operations	No more cynicism
Teamwork; less turf	Teamwork among us
	Harmony among us

How to Construct an Affinity Chart

Following are the eight steps that should be followed when constructing an affinity chart:

1. *Ask.* In a group, ask an open-ended question, even a vague one, that has a wide variety of possible answers or angles to it. Resist any lengthy explanations so that you avoid influencing the range of responses given.

2. *Answer.* The group is then asked to brainstorm responses to the question, with no discussion or evaluation along the way. Joe Colletti of GOAL/QPC[1] suggests setting a "three-word rule," a ground rule that each idea must be stated in a minimum of three words (preferably with a noun and verb included); fewer words may not convey the meaning clearly. For example, without the three-word minimum rule, people might offer thoughts such as "communication," which is very vague. Pushed to use at least three words, they would have to clarify their idea somewhat by saying, "communication of results to staff" or "communication between department heads."

3. *Record.* Ask three people to act as recorders. One person stands at a flip chart and writes down every response given to the question, as quickly as it is generated. The other two people write *each* idea in bold print on a movable sticky note (for example, a 3-by-5-inch Post-it™ note). To prevent the recording process from slowing down the flow of ideas, these two people alternate recording ideas. Listing all the ideas on a flip chart enables the group to see the flow of ideas and avoid duplication. Recording ideas on movable notes is essential to the next step. An alternative is to give group members blank Post-it™ notepads and ask them to write down their ideas as they contribute them. Recorders should record ideas exactly as stated.

4. *Post.* Using a wall you have covered with flip chart paper, ask the two recorders or, if group members recorded their own ideas, the group to help *randomly* post all the ideas on the wall.

5. *Organize.* This next step should be done *without any talking or discussion* so that people can concentrate and assert their own opinions without unnecessary argument over semantics or substance. Ask the group to look for relationships between the ideas, picking up and moving related ideas to form clusters. When using sticky notes, ask people to stick the idea they move onto the idea it relates to (not to the wall) so that the next person to move it will move the entire cluster. During this step, it is important to note the following:
   - Tell the group to resist force-fitting ideas that do not quite belong together.
   - Alert people that there might be "orphans" or "outliers" with no comfortable home. These can form their own cluster.
   - If people disagree about where an item goes, it can be duplicated and put in two places.
   - If your group is so large that not everyone can get close enough to the wall to move the notes, every few minutes ask the people in front to step back and give others a chance.

6. *Name the cluster.* When people feel satisfied with the clusters (which usually takes between 5 and 20 minutes), invite their help in coming up with headers that are descriptive of the elements in that cluster. First, have the group look within the cluster to see whether any one sticky note would make a good header. If they do not identify one, on another sticky note, ideally of a different color, attach a header of their choice to the top of the column of notes that form the cluster. Do not be alarmed at this point if the group wants to break up some clusters because they see components that do not fit. Let them do this until everyone agrees that the clusters make sense.

7. *Relate the clusters.* Sometimes, you can go one step further and move whole clusters so that those that relate to each other are adjacent.

8. *Transfer to paper.* Then or later, transfer your chart to paper. Put solid lines around the clusters and draw lines to connect those clusters that relate to each other.

What happens next depends on your question and purpose. Simple discussion, decision matrices, relationship diagrams, and cause-and-effect diagrams are particularly helpful as alternative follow-up steps:

- *Discussion.* Often simple discussion enables groups to quickly agree on one header as the problem or objective they want to pursue.
- *Decision matrix.* A decision matrix can be used to select one focus for problem solving by rating clusters according to rational criteria (for example, "within our span of influence," "likelihood that we can afford to fix this," and so on).
- *Relationship diagram.* A relationship diagram can be used to identify the headers that, if pursued as objectives, would have the greatest impact on the other headers.
- *Cause-and-effect diagram.* A cause-and-effect diagram can be used to follow up by digging for root causes in which the headers of your affinity chart are used as the names of branches.

Uses of Affinity Charts

When your group feels overwhelmed with ideas or you're having trouble getting a handle on a very vague subject, affinity charts are helpful. For example:

- *If you are trying to solve a problem that has many possible causes.* An affinity chart might lead you to clusters that help identify the roles of the departments contributing to the problem. A next step might be to do a relationship diagram (tool 11) to see which causes are "drivers" and which ones are "results," the drivers being the root causes that, if amenable to change, will have the most powerful impact on the problem.
- *If you are trying to develop a top-priority problem statement about a problem that appears vast and vague.* An affinity chart will help the group to determine more easily how to make their statement of the problem more manageable. A relationship diagram would be effective here, too. Additionally, multivoting or a decision matrix (tool 14) might help your team to select a statement of the problem that is more amenable to change.
- *If you want to set objectives from among a variety of possible choices.*
- *If you want to sift through many possible solutions to a problem.* Looking at the various clusters might help you to explore more easily the related possibilities within each and the advantages and disadvantages of pursuing one cluster over another. A decision matrix is particularly helpful as a follow-up tool. Your group can set criteria for selecting the best cluster of solutions to pursue.
- *If you have brainstormed the tasks involved in implementing an improvement plan and want to organize them into a more manageable framework.*

Here's how one improvement team used affinity charting to develop a statement of mission and values to guide its work. Team members involved everyone and helped them purge their ideas by brainstorming; then, they constructed two affinity charts, one around each of the following questions:

- *What do we want to see as results of our team meetings?* Once it had clusters of related ideas, the team could prioritize them, come up with headers, and make the headers key elements of its mission statement (see figure 11-8 for the brainstorming and resulting two-part affinity chart).

- *What values and behaviors do we want to drive our team?* Once team members had clusters, they could discuss, sort, and make decisions more easily in an effort to develop their mission statement.

The mission statement that resulted from this effort was the following: "Our mission is to institute concrete improvements that lead to heightened customer satisfaction. We will accomplish this in a way that models and reflects the values we place on the professional growth and development of our team members as skilled and optimistic problem solvers."

Benefits of Affinity Charting

Following are some obvious benefits managers will derive from engaging staff in affinity charting:

- Affinity charts are *fun!* They tap a group's creativity by asking people to see relationships or make connections between disparate ideas.
- Affinity charts relieve confusion surrounding questions and issues that have complex, multifaceted answers.
- Affinity charts enable a group to manipulate dozens of ideas in a very short amount of time. The process of sorting through the same number of ideas in a discussion could take hours and leave people feeling confused about the results.
- Affinity charts build group consensus rapidly. Groups tend to feel very proud of themselves because they often reach consensus about the clusters very quickly, without having to listen to meandering discussion.
- The nonverbal nature of the technique sparks participation from everyone, including people who do not usually participate. Also, it reduces the participation of the people who typically dominate.

☐ Tool 11: Relationship Diagrams

Relationship diagrams help individuals and teams to draw logical connections among an array of ideas and identify which ones are drivers and which ones are, at least in part, consequences, results, or subsequent events affected by the drivers.

For example, let's consider the problem of a team that has evidence of a morale problem and wants to tackle it. Because *morale* is a big, very vague problem, the team must develop a statement of the problem that makes it manageable. Members must brainstorm reasons for the problem and then create an affinity chart to organize those reasons or causes into clusters so they can identify one important root cause. The affinity chart (see figure 11-9) will highlight the major causes of the morale problem, which will thus help the team to focus on one cause for its improvement effort.

This is where the relationship diagram comes in. Team members arrange all the headers on a wipe-off board or a flip chart in no particular order, as shown in section A of figure 11-10 (p. 159). Then, the manager or other facilitator asks the team to consider every *pair* of headers and determine whether, for that pair, A drives B, B drives A, or neither. If A drives B, an arrow is drawn from A to B to show this relationship. However, a relationship between items is not required. In many cases, no arrows are drawn because the team does not see a strong logical or directional relationship. After methodically checking for a relationship between A and any other item and then between B and any other item, the team ends up with a relationship diagram (similar to the one in section B of figure 11-10), referred to by some as a spaghetti diagram for obvious reasons.

Next, team members count the number of arrows leading *from* each item and write this number near that item. The items with the highest numbers are the powerhouse

Figure 11-9. Affinity Chart to Determine Causes of a Morale Problem

Ineffective, Unfair Supervisors	Lack of Recognition	Employees Not Involved or Valued
They don't tell us things Information vacuum They play favorites Poor role models Authoritarian; treat us like kids	Low pay No merit pay Risk taking is punished No response to our ideas We're taken for granted	Authoritarian supervisors Good ideas ignored No interest in our opinions No forums for input "We–they" antagonism Administration doesn't tell truth
Co-Worker Friction	**Frustrating Systems/Problems**	**Employee Burnout/Fatigue**
Tension with peers Some don't do job Jealousies in team Endless griping Supervisor doesn't intervene	Cumbersome systems Lack of tools to do job, but "do it anyway" Short-staffing Staff takes flack for poor systems Administration uses band-aids, not solutions Problems go on year after year	Overwork Staff shortages Too many priorities Crisis-driven managers; fires to put out

items, the drivers or root causes that, if addressed, would have a ripple effect on other elements of the global morale problem. In this case, A ("ineffective, unfair supervisors") was the item with the most outward-bound arrows (four); B, C, and E each had two, D had one, and F had none.

As a result, the team decided to focus its improvement effort on the quality of supervision. Members decided that the supervisors in their organization either had not been adequately trained or had not been expected to be leaders who set high standards, involve staff, share information openly, and identify and pursue systems problems that interfere with their staff's ability to do their jobs. The team believed that if the quality of supervision were addressed and dramatically upgraded, this would have a powerful, positive impact on every other contributor to the overall morale problem.

How to Construct a Relationship Diagram

Before constructing a relationship diagram, you need to select several elements, objectives, or actions that you now want to causally or chronologically relate to one another. You can derive such a list of elements through conducting discussions, brainstorming, or developing an affinity chart.

The following four steps should be followed in constructing a relationship diagram:

1. *Arrange headings in a circle.* Label the headings A, B, C, and so on.
2. *Draw relationship arrows.* Starting with A and working around the circle, draw directional arrows showing perceived relationships between all the headings. Don't force relationships that are not clear. If there is disagreement among group members about whether a relationship exists or about the direction of the relationship,

take that as a sign that the relationship is not clear and do not connect the two ideas.

3. *Count the number of arrows leaving each item.* Then write that number next to the item.

4. *Draw conclusions.* If there is an item that drives several others, and *if* that header is amenable to change, it would be a logical focus for further exploration. It has the power of a root cause because positive change within it will, in turn, relieve several other symptoms.

Figure 11-10. The Relationship Diagram Drawn from Affinity Chart in Figure 11-9

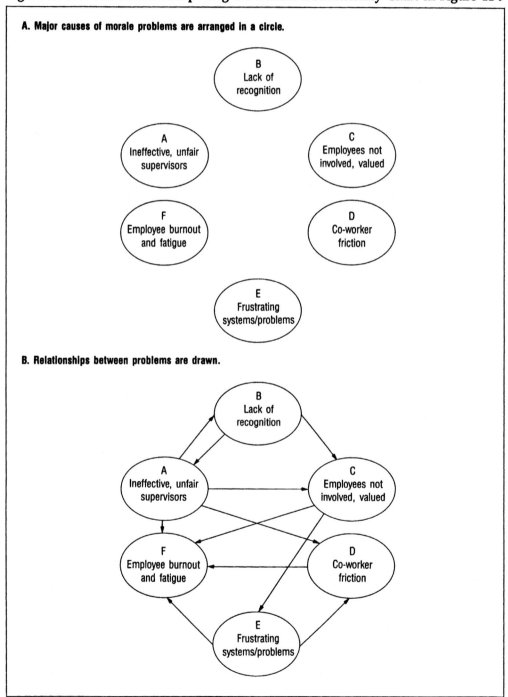

A. Major causes of morale problems are arranged in a circle.

B. Relationships between problems are drawn.

Uses of Relationship Diagrams

Relationship diagrams help you to causally or chronologically relate several discrete concepts or actions. Finding these relationships is especially helpful in identifying root causes or objectives for improvement and sequencing actions that are key to implementing solutions. More specifically, they are used to:

- Sort out the relationships among numerous complex ideas.
- Identify problems, forces, or causes that, if alleviated, would have major effects.
- Separate symptoms from causes, identifying the root causes that drive the symptoms.
- Create a tree diagram that sequences the tasks or elements in your implementation plan, starting with the prerequisite (or driving) tasks.
- Work in combination with force-field analysis. In force-field analysis, you identify driving and restraining forces affecting your ability to reach your goal. A relationship diagram is used to sort out these driving forces by comparing them and identifying the select few that have the greatest influence on the others. The goal is to identify the causal or most influential force so that you can focus your resources on the few forces that, if altered, would have the most far-reaching ripple effects.

☐ Tool 12: Cause-and-Effect Diagrams

Cause-and-effect diagrams help to identify and illustrate the relationships between an effect, an outcome, or a problem and hunches about the possible causes or factors that contribute to it. The purpose is to articulate theories about root causes and see relationships among them so that you can consciously select those deserving further attention. These diagrams are also sometimes called Ishikawa diagrams (for their founder, Kaora Ishikawa, Tokyo, 1950), fishbone diagrams (because of their shape), and "fishykawa" diagrams (a combination of both). A generic cause-and-effect diagram is shown in figure 11-11 and a fishbone diagram is shown in figure 11-12.

Cause-and-effect diagrams are multileveled. Level 1 asks what are the causes of the effect? Level 2 asks what causes each of these causes? Or, what are the "subsidiary" causes? Level 3 asks what causes these subsidiary causes? And so on until the root causes are exposed. The root causes tend to be the causes at the lowest level, those that are concrete, those that are directly controllable, and when reduced or eliminated, those that relieve the problem. A cause-and-effect diagram with three levels is shown in figure 11-13 (p. 162).

How to Construct a Cause-and-Effect Diagram

Before developing a cause-and-effect diagram, you need to clarify your problem or effect so that you can focus your thinking about its possible causes. Through brainstorming, you might also have generated possible causes that you now wish to organize and crystallize. Following are the steps involved in constructing a cause-and-effect diagram:

1. *Summarize your problem statement.* Write your problem statement in as few words as possible in a box at the pointed end of a long arrow, the so-called spine of the fish (see section A of figure 11-13).
2. *Determine the headers.* These are the categories you want to use to trigger thinking about possible causes (between three and six categories). Connect these to the spine with arrows (called bones or branches), as shown in section B of figure 11-13.
   - Use these versatile categories to trigger possible causes of the effect you're trying to improve.

Figure 11-11. Generic Cause-and-Effect Diagram

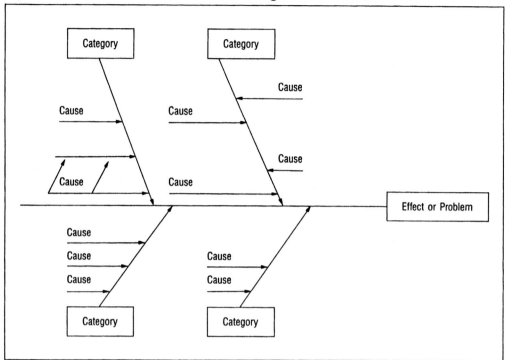

Figure 11-12. Fishbone Diagram

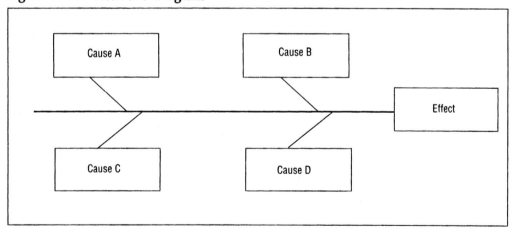

- Ishikawa suggested using generic headers such as material, machine, measurement, man (people), methods. Other generic possibilities include:
  - Equipment, people, materials, methods, money
  - Policies, people, paper, technology, methods
- You can also make up your own headers to fit your problem. For instance, to explore possible causes for dissatisfaction among one of your customer groups (for example, patients), you could use these headers: technical competence, people skills, amenities, systems/processes, environment, cost.
3. *Determine what elements of each category are contributing to the effect.* These elements are the subsidiary causes that influence the effect in question. Write those answers on lines or bones branching off the category lines (see section C of figure 11-13).

Figure 11-13. Construction of a Cause-and-Effect Diagram

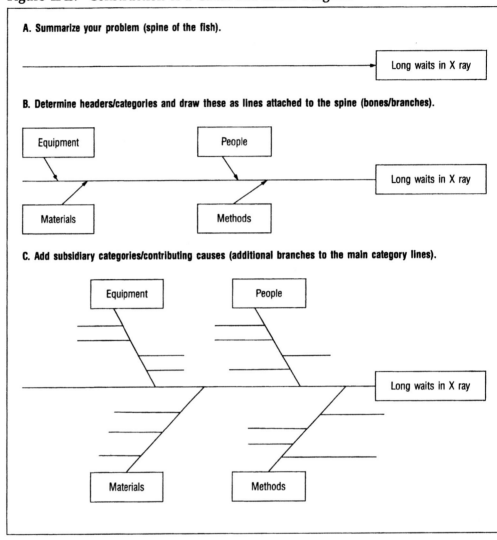

A. Summarize your problem (spine of the fish).

Long waits in X ray

B. Determine headers/categories and draw these as lines attached to the spine (bones/branches).

Equipment   People

Long waits in X ray

Materials   Methods

C. Add subsidiary categories/contributing causes (additional branches to the main category lines).

Equipment   People

Long waits in X ray

Materials   Methods

4. *Continue to dig for the causes of the causes in each branch of your chart until you reach what you believe to be the root cause of each bone.* A good rule of thumb is to ask why five times to ferret out root causes.

5. *Clean out the diagram before testing the theories reflected within it.* Because brainstorming is used along the way and it produces freewheeling thinking, not all the causes generated will turn out to be pertinent. Thus, the logic for each cause should be checked. For each set of bones, work both forward and backward to double-check the validity of the causal links.

6. *Narrow down your theories.* To accomplish this, use methods such as the following:
   • Show the chart to people close to the causes identified and invite their views about the most powerful ones.
   • Vote to select key causes worthy of further investigation. Give people several votes each; then narrow down the list and vote again among the winners.
   • Give every group member 10 points to allocate to causes as he or she sees fit. This enables people to numerically express intense beliefs about certain key causes. (If they wish, they may give all their points to one cause or divide them among several causes.) Add up the numbers and explore the winners first.
   • Do a relationship diagram (tool 11) to help you select those with positive ripple effects.

- Rule out the causes that you believe are not amenable to change, in other words, those over which you have no control.
- Once you've narrowed these down to a manageable number, collect data to test your theories about causes. The result could be expressed in a Pareto chart (see chapter 10, tool 6).

Figure 11-14 is an example of a cause-and-effect diagram used by Holston Valley Hospital and Medical Center, in Kingsport, Tennessee, to determine the causes of time delays from the point a decision is made to admit a patient from the emergency department to the point the patient arrives at an inpatient room. The problem statement for this diagram was: "Reduction of time from emergency department to bed." As can be seen, the

Figure 11-14. Sample Cause-and-Effect Diagram

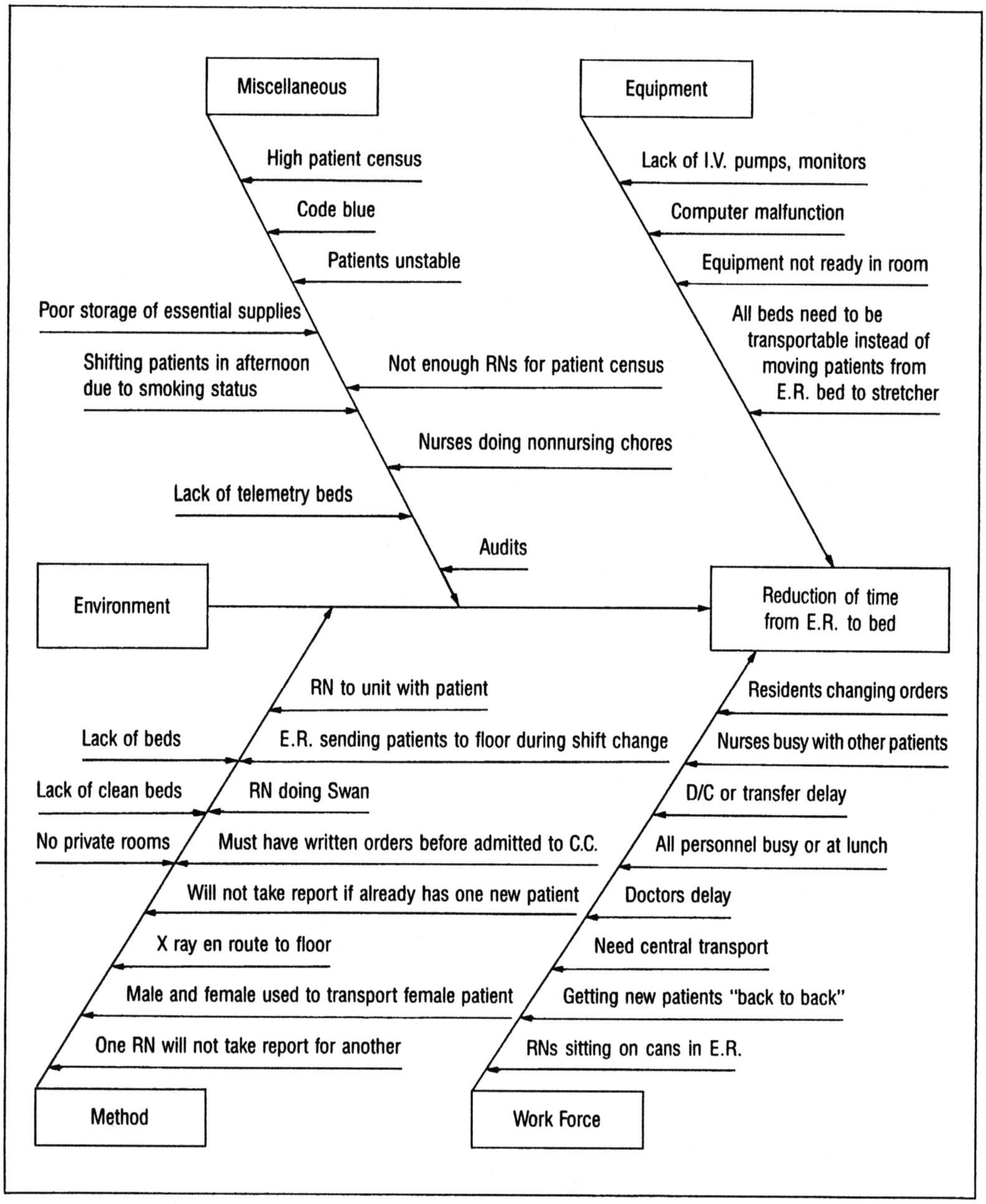

Reprinted, with permission, from Holston Valley Hospital and Medical Center, Kingsport, TN, 1990.

163

headers selected to trigger brainstorming of causes are "miscellaneous," "equipment," "environment," "method," and "work force." These headers comprise level one of the diagram. Then within each header, the team brainstormed subsidiary causes to make this a level-two diagram. Afterward, team members asked themselves, "Which elements are causal?"

Process Cause-and-Effect Diagrams: A Variation

After flowcharting a process, you can create a cause-and-effect diagram to generate possible causes of problems *within and between steps*. For example, consider the simplified process that has resulted in late medication delivery to patients, as shown in the flowchart in figure 11-15. A cause-and-effect diagram can be constructed to identify the causes of problems between and within steps that are resulting in delays. The simple diagram in figure 11-16 illustrates sources of delay between the time medications are delivered to the unit and the time they are delivered to the patient.

Uses of Cause-and-Effect Diagrams

Cause-and-effect diagrams are mainly used to search for root causes of problems. The following are some specific uses:

- To help team members generate and articulate their theories about causes by providing a simple, straightforward, and enjoyable structure for productive brainstorming.
- To sift through and organize the brainstormed items within the basic categories and verify that important possible causes were not omitted.

Figure 11-15. Flowchart of Process of Medication Delivery to Patients

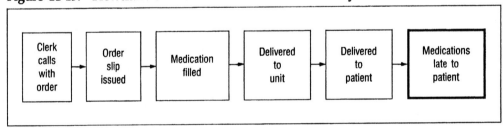

Figure 11-16. Process Cause-and-Effect Diagram

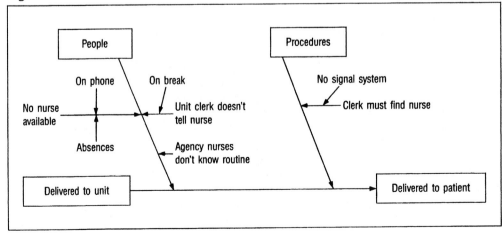

- To dig for solutions to problems. Place a goal instead of a problem in the "effect" box and then use the cause-and-effect diagram to brainstorm approaches to this goal. This helps you to find powerful solutions.

Precautions and Tips

Take note of the following before working with cause-and-effect diagrams:

- Make sure everyone in the group agrees on the problem statement before you begin.
- Involve people close to all aspects of the problem so that your pool of possible causes is comprehensive and real.
- Do not think you are doing a sloppy job if some causes appear on more than one bone of your chart. Multiple relationships often show up on cause-and-effect diagrams.
- Don't give up. Cause-and-effect diagrams can become very complex. The answers are in the details. Rather than abandoning the technique as it becomes complex, move each major bone to its own sheet of paper, where you will have more space to develop it fully.

☐ Tool 13: Force-Field Analysis

To produce improvement or move toward a goal, you have to challenge the status quo. You can do this in two ways: You can (1) strengthen the forces that are currently pushing performance upward (the driving forces) or (2) weaken or eliminate the forces that are impeding improved performance (the restraining forces). This is the logic that underlies force-field analysis.

When you want to tackle a problem or goal, it helps to start by examining the forces that are contributing to the status quo, or the current situation. These include opposing forces that create a balance, a static force field or frozen condition. Change happens when one type of force overwhelms another. Performance *deteriorates* when restraining forces overpower driving forces, in other words, when restraining forces inhibit or block improvement or solutions. Performance *improves* when driving forces overpower restraining forces, in other words, when driving forces push toward, encourage, or support improvement or solutions.

The following example will illustrate how force-field charts are used. A large midwestern hospital conducted an interdepartmental services survey in which each department rated every other department on service dimensions. As it turned out, the education department received a very low satisfaction score on its provision of audiovisual support services. These services included purchase, maintenance, delivery, setup, pickup, and technical support of a variety of audiovisual equipment used by physicians, in-service educators, administrators, and other hospital staff in educational programs, grand rounds, meetings, and conferences.

With the survey results in hand, the department manager decided to organize a team to focus on improving internal customer satisfaction with audiovisual support services. She formed a team consisting of her staff and conducted a force-field analysis. The goal was to achieve 100 percent satisfaction with the department's audiovisual support services. The manager asked the team, "What forces are currently operating that contribute positively to our customers' satisfaction with our services? What are the driving forces?" Then she asked, "What forces are working against or impeding satisfaction among our customers? What are the restraining forces?" The resulting force-field chart is shown in figure 11-17.

The manager recognized that if restraining forces remained as strong or stronger than driving forces, customer satisfaction would not improve. However, she also knew that

Figure 11-17. Force-Field Chart for Education Department of a Hospital

Current Level	
0% Satisfaction	**100% Satisfaction**
Driving Forces	**Restraining Forces**
Talented audiovisual staff	No backup staff
Location convenient to meeting rooms	Customers want hand-holding
Beeper provides access	Growing demand
Increasing number of VCRs available	Old equipment; no features
Some people don't expect much from us	No maintenance contracts
Extra bulbs with all projectors	Lean budget
Customers get service free	No written instructions on equipment; makes people dependent
Pressure from survey results to make improvements	No lighting controls in conference rooms
Scrutiny from administration	Phone requests met with impatience to make improvements
	No feedback device
	No periodic assessment of customer needs
	Because no charge, people order "just in case"
	Long-term employees; used to how we do things

if a restraining force could be reduced or a driving force strengthened, a net improvement in internal customer satisfaction would be likely to result. Through discussion and rank-ordering, the team reached agreement on the most powerful restraining and driving forces, specifically those amenable to change, and created a plan for altering those forces so that service would improve and, as a result, customer satisfaction would increase.

Force-field analysis is a format you can use to help a group identify and think through the forces that influence an improvement they want to make. You will be more successful if you consider the counterforces as well as the forces working to support the change. Once these forces are made explicit, the group can discuss the relative intensity and priority of the forces on both sides of the ledger. And by understanding counterforces, the group can develop contingency responses to be used, if necessary, during implementation. The results guide the group toward effective strategy decisions.

How to Construct a Force-Field Analysis

Following are the basic steps in the construction of a force-field analysis:

1. Clearly define the improvement you are planning and write it down as a goal statement at the upper right-hand side of a sheet of paper so that the group can continuously focus on it.
2. Across the top of a large sheet of paper, draw a horizontal line representing the continuum of performance related to your goal:

    0% —————————————————————————— 100%

3. Represent the current performance level or status quo by a vertical line down the middle of the page.

    0% ————————————————|———————————— 100%

4. Without initial analysis, brainstorm first the driving forces and then the restraining forces that affect this performance level. List the driving forces on the left under an arrow pointing in the direction of the performance level. List the restraining forces on the right under an arrow pointing backward, illustrating that the performance level is being held back.

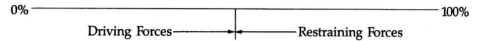

5. Narrow down your lists to include only those forces that have the greatest potential to help you reach your objective. Select three or four driving forces that group members think they can realistically strengthen and an equal number of restraining forces they believe can be weakened. Affinity charting can be used to sort through and cluster the forces on each side of the chart. In this case, voting may be a useful method for narrowing down your lists. An option is to use a decision matrix (tool 14) to help you employ rational criteria for judging among your alternatives and picking your preference. For example, using a decision matrix, have everyone rate your six to eight possibilities according to, first, each one's strength or potential impact if changed and, second, your ability to influence it.

Following is an example of how an improvement team in one hospital used force-field analysis to confront the problem of not enough word-processing operators. Upon analysis, team members discovered that most departments had one person who did the lion's share of word processing, whereas other work loads varied tremendously. After considering a variety of possible solutions, the team decided to think through the development of a centralized word-processing center that would require the transfer into one department of several word-processing operators now located in various departments. The team's force-field analysis is shown in figure 11-18. Upon further discussion of the potential impact and malleability of the various forces, team members decided to address one driving force and four restraining forces in their implementation plan (see figure 11-19).

Uses of Force-Field Analysis

Generally, force-field analysis helps a group of people to quickly generate and display factors or forces that have an impact on their achievement of a particular objective. Following are some specific uses of force-field analysis:

Figure 11-18. Force-Field Analysis for Creating a Central Word-Processing Department

Current Level	
0%	100% Effective
Driving Forces	**Restraining Forces**
Greater efficiency	Breakup of work groups
Less slack time of nonbusy departments	Managers' fear of losing control
Less stress for processors in busiest departments	Employees' fear of layoffs
Greater expertise from "specialists"	Department-based people do *more* than word processing; other duties abandoned
Professional manager would raise standards	Managers' fear of favoritism by administrators
"New look"	"No one will get to know our work"

- To identify improvement opportunities. For example, let's say you track customer satisfaction and are dissatisfied with your results. You can do a force-field analysis for each of your customer's main requirements, as shown in figure 11-20.
- To identify key causes that, if altered, would have a positive impact on a solution to a problem. For example, if the problem identified were too many medication errors, you could then ask the following questions: "Which forces are restraining error-free medication (untrained staff, too much pressure on pharmacists, inconsistent supervision, unclear handwriting on orders, keystroke errors in computer, and so forth)? Which forces are driving error-free medication (consistent quality checks, checklists for common medications, and so forth)?"
- To evaluate the likelihood that a new program or proposed improvement would actually reap the intended benefits. For example, will placement of computers in our medical staff's offices strengthen physicians' loyalty to our hospital?
- To help think through a realistic implementation plan that includes countermeasures designed to diminish restraining forces or barriers, as well as strategies to capitalize on driving forces.

Figure 11-19. Implementation Plan Resulting from Force-Field Analysis in Figure 11-18

Driving Force	Strategies to Strengthen
Professional manager would raise standards	Presentation to department heads should spell out how department will be managed: • To improve quality of output • To make explicit work-flow system to assure every manager that his or her work will be done by deadline • To train and coach people to higher skill level

Restraining Forces	Strategies to Minimize
Breakup of work groups	Fund and run team building for new people in new department; help them "bond"
Managers' fear of losing control	Make explicit the new department's system for meeting *every* manager's deadlines
Employees' fear of layoffs	Create and publicize clear policy about no layoffs, only transfers
Secretaries in departments do more than word process	Create minimum level of support for departments in need
"No one will get to know our work"	Assign each pool member to specific group of departments with "first right of refusal" on their work

Figure 11-20. Example of a Force-Field Analysis Form for Each Customer Requirement

Customer Requirement	What's driving?	What's impeding?
#1		
#2		
#3		

☐ Tool 14: Decision Matrices

A *decision matrix* is an evaluation tool that helps you to compare and choose among alternative problems or solutions in a rational way. Once you have generated alternatives (problems, possible causes, or solutions), a decision matrix helps you to select the best choice. It enables you to quickly profile every group member's views about the relative strengths and weaknesses of alternatives and graphically see the extent of consensus or disagreement. By involving everyone in this rational approach, you will reduce lengthy discussions and save substantial amounts of time and at the same time build consensus and confidence in your ultimate decision.

In improvement teams, group members often lean toward one alternative or another without having a clear reason for their preference. Do people select one alternative over another because of cost, ease of implementation, politics, likelihood of increasing customer satisfaction, time involved, expected acceptance of key players, the cost of *not* doing it, or some other reason? This technique helps team members to make their criteria *explicit*, which makes it easier for them to apply their shared criteria in the evaluation of alternatives and to choose among them.

Most teams also find it easier and quicker to reach consensus on appropriate criteria for choosing among alternatives than to reach consensus by discussing alternative by alternative. By focusing first on criteria, team members then have a shared philosophy they can apply in making their decision. Figure 11-21 is a basic template for a decision matrix.

How to Construct a Decision Matrix

Following are the basic steps involved in constructing a decision matrix:

1. Select criteria for evaluating your alternatives. The team should spend as much time as necessary to agree on criteria because these criteria are the guiding principles by which you will evaluate alternatives.
2. Write the criteria (impact, cost of unmet expectations, cost of implementation, wear and tear on staff, and so forth) in the boxes along the top of a matrix chart.
3. Decide on the relative *weight* of each criterion. Are some criteria twice as important as others? If so, the more important criterion receives a higher weight, or multiplier, (for example, 2) and the less important receives a lower weight (for example, 1). If the criteria are equally important, they are weighted the same.

Figure 11-21. Basic Template for a Decision Matrix

Alternatives	Criteria / Weight					Total	Rank

4. List the alternative problems or solutions in the left-hand column.
5. Have each person in the group independently rate each alternative according to each criterion and fill out his or her matrix, writing a 1, 2, or 3 in each box opposite the alternatives and below the criteria, as each sees fit:

$$1 = \text{low rating}$$
$$2 = \text{medium rating}$$
$$3 = \text{high rating}$$

An option is to use a rank-ordering system. For instance, if the group is considering five alternatives, each member compares all alternatives against one criterion at a time, rank-ordering the alternatives. This forces people to choose among alternatives, making trade-offs instead of giving every alternative a high score.
6. Have each person total his or her score for each row by multiplying the rating in each box by the weight assigned to the numbers in that column. On the right, people should have a total score for each alternative.
7. Tally the scores by adding up all group members' scores for each alternative.
8. Summarize the results by listing the alternatives from high to low.
9. Use the results to reach a decision. Look at the top-rated alternatives and discuss them further. If the results do not ring true with people, ask, "Have we omitted an important criterion?" If so, alter your criteria and redo your ratings until the group feels that the results provide a sound basis for decision making.

Uses of Decision Matrices

Decision matrices are used to do the following:

• To select among alternative problems
• To select among alternative causes
• To select among alternative countermeasures or solutions
• To select among alternative implementation steps

Figures 11-21 (without weighting) and 11-22 (with weighting) are two examples of decision matrices. The matrix in figure 11-22 was created because patients and families were complaining about unclear, incomplete discharge instructions. The goal was to have 90 percent of patients and families perceive discharge instructions as clear and complete. In this matrix, the lower score was the better one. With the results in hand, the group ruled out idea number 2 and then created additional criteria that they felt would differentiate between the two remaining options; the new criteria were "speed of implementation" and "likely impact on patient/family satisfaction." The problem resulting in the matrix in figure 11-23 was how to best and most quickly communicate important news to all employees. A third type of decision matrix is the one shown in figure 11-24 (p. 172). This matrix is used to select among alternative solutions or projects by applying the relevant criteria (for example, cost to implement, time involved, return on investment, anticipated resistance, and so forth).

Figure 11-22. Decision Matrix: How to Clarify Discharge Instructions for Patients

Alternative Solutions	Criteria			Total	Rank
	Cost-Effective	User-Friendly	Convenient for Staff		
Rewrite instructions/ checklist for major diagnostic categories	1	2	2	5	2
Produce videos for major diagnosis	3	3	3	9	3
Hire nurses to do follow-up calls	2	1	1	4	1

Figure 11-23. Decision Matrix: How to Best Communicate Important News to Employees

Alternatives	Criteria/Weight											
	1 = High 10 = Low			1 = Low 10 = High			1 = Hard 10 = Easy			1 = Long 10 = Short		
	Cost (× 2)			Acceptability			Ease of Implementation			Time Involved		
	Rating weight subtotal			Rating weight subtotal			Rating weight subtotal			Rating weight subtotal		Total	Rank
Mail to employee's home	1	2	2	5	1	5	3	1	3	3	1	3	13	3
Insert in paycheck	3	2	6	8	1	8	5	1	5	8	1	8	27	2
Post around hospital	6	2	12	3	1	3	8	1	8	4	1	4	27	2
Special feature on intercom	10	2	20	3	1	3	10	1	10	4	1	4	37	1

Figure 11-24. Decision Matrix Used to Select among Alternative Solutions or Projects

Problems	Impact on Customer Satisfaction	× Employee Impact	× Need for Improvement	= Total
1				
2				
3				
4				
5				
6				
7				

SCALE: 1 = none   2 = somewhat   3 = moderate   4 = very   5 = extreme

Precautions

- Focus up front on your primary goal. If the group doesn't agree on the overall goal or results you want to achieve, you are much more likely to have conflict in your approaches because people will be focusing on different goals or dimensions of the problem.
- The results of using a decision matrix are only as good as the quality and relevance of the criteria you select. Be sure to select your criteria carefully before your group completes the matrix.
- Suspend criticism until you have generated an array of possibilities. If you let people judge one another's ideas before you have generated a healthy set of alternatives, creativity and fluency of idea generation are stifled. Be strict about urging people to hold criticism or any evaluation of ideas until the team has generated the full array.
- If your results bother you, trust your instincts. Sometimes, a team will undergo a thorough problem-solving process and feel that it has to live with the result even if the result goes against the team's instincts. A decision matrix merely helps you to consider alternatives using a rational approach. Its worth, however, depends on the quality of your criteria. If your team's output does not ring true, stop and discuss this observation. Such discussion tends to lead to breakthrough insights about the problem and what it *really* takes to solve it. In other words, techniques are designed to trigger new levels of thinking about the problem. It's that thinking, not the techniques themselves, that leads to quality solutions. So trust your instincts and do not let any techniques constrain you.
- Acknowledge that some solutions are simple and some are not. The overworked receptionist might need a more comfortable chair, more frequent and shorter breaks, a backup for when multiple phones are ringing, hardware that works 100 percent of the time, and a vacation. Many problems require a combination of actions. Do not give in to simple, one-dimensional answers when your wisdom

tells you that there is more to it than that. So with a decision matrix, if *no* alternatives really score high, keep at it.

☐ Tool 15: Tree Diagrams

A *tree diagram* is an extremely versatile way to show graphically the breakdown of large questions, goals, or problems into their increasingly more detailed elements. These diagrams help you to move from general to specific in an organized fashion, showing the logical connections that led you there. (Figure 11-25 shows the basic format of a tree diagram.)

How to Construct a Tree Diagram

Following are the basic steps involved in developing a tree diagram:

1. *Clarify your purpose.*
   - If you want to find root causes, ask why.
   - If you want to generate alternatives, ask how.
   - If you want to clarify an idea or break it down into its elements, ask what do we mean by this and what are its components.
2. *Generate alternative causes, tactics, or tasks related to your core statement, goal, or idea.* Some teams brainstorm these alternatives and record them on a flip chart before they organize them, select among them, and place them on a tree diagram. Others record each item on cards or Post-it™ notes so that the items can be immediately manipulated and arranged appropriately on the tree.
3. *Evaluate your ideas and narrow them down to a manageable number.* An easy way to evaluate your ideas is to have every team member code each element as either "feasible," "don't know until we have more information," or "impossible." After polling the results, you need to reach consensus on the elements you want to place at the second level of your tree.

Figure 11-25. Basic Format of the Tree Diagram

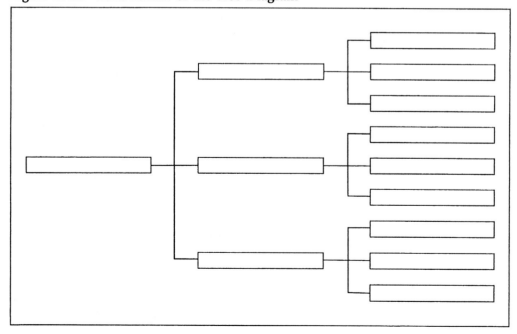

4. *Construct your tree.*
- Level One. Write your overall goal, concept, or idea on the left side of a wallboard or flip chart, or work on a table using notecards. If you are working on a flip chart or wallboard, use Post-it™ notes to record the elements. These can be easily manipulated without having to redraw your entire chart. Remind people of the why, how, and what questions that need to be asked to move you to the next stage.
- Level Two. Working on one step at a time, write the answers to your why, how, or what questions on parallel lines or branches that connect to the stem.
- Level Three. Focusing on one level-two element at a time, break down each into sublevels. Go through the same process for additional levels if needed, checking the logic in your tree diagram by moving from right to left. At your most detailed level, ask, "Does this lead us up the tree?" Fill in gaps and remove illogical or unrelated items.

Uses of Tree Diagrams

Tree diagrams are highly versatile tools for organizing related or chronological elements or actions. Following are some typical uses of the tree diagram in quality improvement:

- *To identify root causes.* Because tree diagrams are often used as an alternative to cause-and-effect diagrams, some people call them "why–why" or "five-whys" diagrams. *Five whys* refers to the five levels of answers to the why question that are recommended. Figure 11-26 is an example of a simple why–why diagram.
- *To generate alternatives.* Tree diagrams are often used to generate alternative solutions or countermeasures. This variation is sometimes referred to as a how–how diagram. Figure 11-27 is an example of a how–how diagram.
- *To evaluate countermeasures.* The countermeasures tree diagram (combined with a decision matrix) enables you to see relationships between your problem and possible solutions and then to evaluate the possible solutions against several criteria in order to make a decision. Countermeasures are tactics aimed at alleviating the root causes—the what. *Practical methods* are the specific tasks needed to institute the countermeasures—the how. Figure 11-28 (p. 176) is an example of a countermeasures tree diagram.
- *To tell an improvement story.* Tree diagrams can also be used to tell an improvement story by showing the unfolding of your understanding of a problem, the method of verification, the countermeasures you have decided to take, and the actions needed to institute those countermeasures. Figure 11-29 (p. 177) shows a countermeasures tree diagram used to illustrate an improvement story.
- *To clarify ideas.* Tree diagrams are also used to clarify fuzzy ideas or goals, fleshing out their multiple elements so that they are no longer fuzzy. For example, consider the goal of improving systems that affect physician satisfaction. What systems? What is meant by this? A tree diagram can be used to help a group break down the general into the specific or the abstract into the operational so that the group becomes clear about what it is investigating. See figure 11-30 (p. 178) for an example of this type of diagram.
- *To generate a plan.* Probably the most common use of tree diagrams is to map out an implementation plan (described in a later section).
- *To take stock of what is currently being done related to a goal.* This use of a tree diagram enables you to identify gaps.
- *To create a contingency plan in the face of anticipated obstacles.* A tree diagram of the type sometimes called a process–decision–program chart[2] helps you to organize your approach to obstacles that you think might occur as you implement a plan. For each step in your plan, ask, "What might go wrong here?" Level two of your tree diagram shows these possibilities. Then, at level three, specify the actions you can take to prevent or correct each obstacle or minimize its effect (figure 11-31, p. 178).

Figure 11-26. Example of a Why–Why Tree Diagram

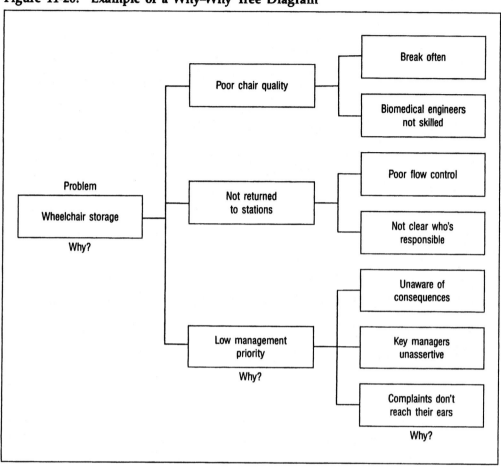

Figure 11-27. Example of a How–How Tree Diagram

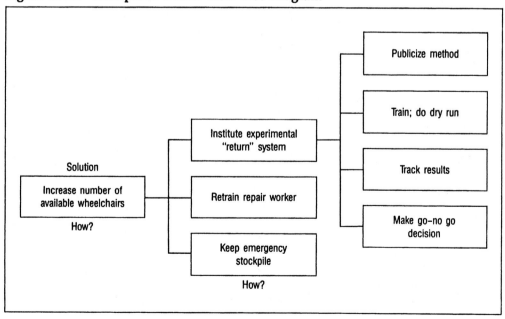

Figure 11-28. Countermeasures Tree Diagram and Decision Matrix

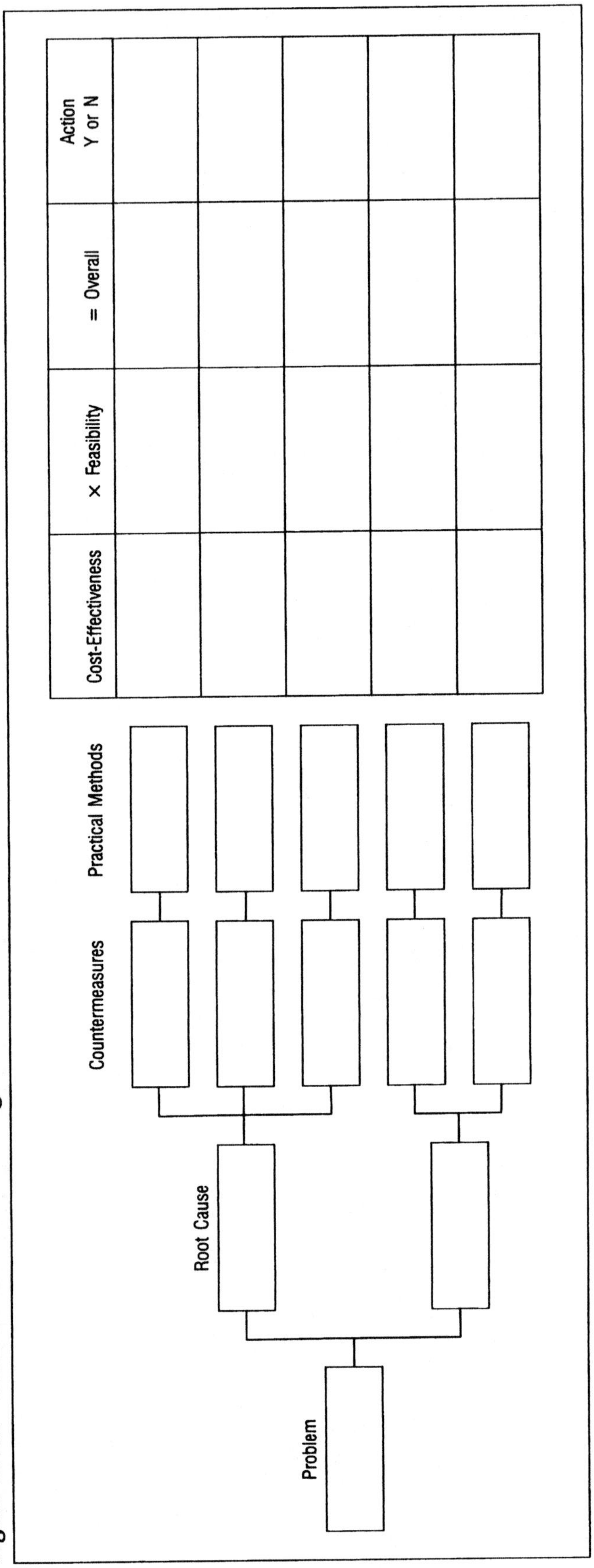

Figure 11-29. Countermeasures Tree Diagram to Illustrate an Improvement

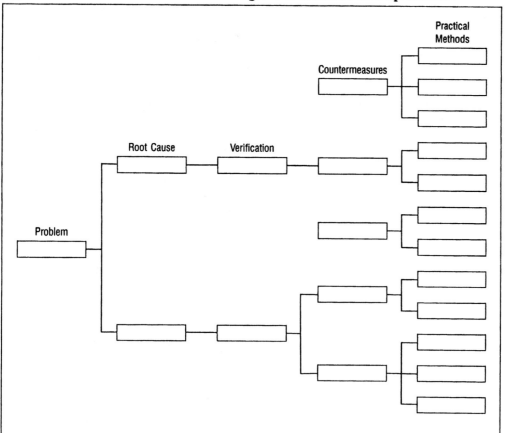

Tips

The following tips may be helpful in selecting your tools:

- Many people prefer tree diagrams to cause-and-effect diagrams because their linear nature makes them easier to complete and read.
- You can use affinity charts and relationship diagrams to generate your main goals or tactics and then flesh out the details with a tree diagram.

Figure 11-30. Tree Diagram Used to Clarify Ideas

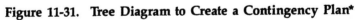

Systems that affect physician satisfaction	Admissions	Efficiency	
		Communication	
		Courtesy	
	Discharge	Speed	
		Nursing support	
		Transport	
	Auxiliary scheduling	Timeliness	
		Patient access when physician visits	
		Appropriate sequencing	
	Results	Radiology	Timeliness
			Accuracy
			Interpretation
			Readability
		Lab	Accurate
			Complete
			Timeliness
			Readability
	Billing	Accuracy	
		Courtesy when complaint	
		Timeliness	
	Communication with administration	Responsiveness to complaints	
		Sharing of information	
		Systems for involving doctors in decisions	

Figure 11-31. Tree Diagram to Create a Contingency Plan*

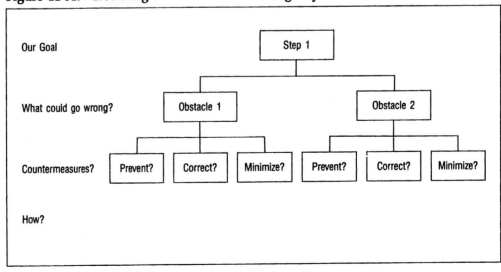

*Sometimes called a process-decision-program chart.

☐ Tool 16: Action Planning

Needless to say, a brilliant solution or improvement idea is not enough; it has to become a reality. You need to involve the right people in accepting the idea and doing their part to implement it. In other words, you need an *action plan*, a plan that includes the steps to be taken, the people/departments responsible for each step, a time frame for each step's implementation, how you will follow up to ensure that the steps were taken, and how you will check for results. This plan must be implemented with the people responsible for translating the improvement into practice.

Action-planning tools help you to draw a blueprint for your plan so that all key players share their understanding of what is supposed to happen in considerable detail. The tools are variations on several of the other tools presented earlier in this book.

Key Steps in Action Planning

Following are the essential steps in the action-planning process:

1. State the end result that would signify a significant improvement or enhancement to your process.
2. Identify the actions needed to achieve the result (perhaps by brainstorming) and the resources needed to complete each action.
3. Put these steps in sequential order (for example, in a flowchart), at times allowing for parallel or concurrent actions.
4. Identify anticipated problems and how you plan to prevent or handle them.
5. Assign responsibilities and set performance expectations.
6. Determine the deadline for completing the overall plan and the start-to-finish dates for each step.
7. Identify your methods for monitoring implementation and intended and unintended effects—in time for corrective action. Identify indicators; figure out the hows, whos, and whens for using them; and plan on checkpoints for when the right people will review and act on the data.
8. Decide who, if anyone, must approve your plan before implementation.

Tools for Action Planning

The tools described in the following sections are: work sheets for plan implementation, guides for making your case, Gantt charts, work sheets for anticipating problems, tree diagrams for action planning, and storyboards.

Work Sheets: Tools for Planning Implementation of an Improvement
The work sheet shown in figure 11-32 can be used as a guide for planning implementation of an improvement idea. It helps to ask the questions that are central to developing a thorough and clear plan. Many teams complete this work sheet and transfer their decisions to a tree diagram or Gantt chart that then becomes their implementation road map.

Guide for Making Your Case
Once you have developed your plan, you very likely have to sell it, first to yourself or your team and then to all the people who will play a role in making it happen. Figure 11-33 presents a guide that can be used to help your team work out a thorough and effective case for acquiring whatever approval or resources you need to turn your plan into reality.

Figure 11-32. Work Sheet: Tool for Planning Implementation of an Improvement

Objective: _____

_____

Possible obstacles: _____

_____

Preventive steps: _____

_____

Key steps to ensure successful implementation: Who? When? _____

_____

Review and assessment: Who? How? When? _____

_____

Benefits/expected results/potential impact: _____

_____

Actual results (to be completed later): _____

_____

Figure 11-33. Guide for Making Your Case

1. The problem
2. The solution
3. Why this solution? Justification
4. Projected impact/benefits for
   - customers
   - organization
   - staff
   - financial status
5. The risks and costs involved
   - Customer impact
   - Staff impact (training, receptivity, staffing levels)
   - Tools, equipment needs
   - Dollars
   - Time
6. How and why the potential benefits outweigh the costs
7. Implementation plan
   - What?
   - How?
   - Where?
   - When?
   - Who?
8. What barriers are expected, and what will be done about them?

Gantt Charts

Gantt charts are horizontal bar charts that show the time relationship among steps in an implementation plan. Along the left side of the chart are the steps in the plan. Along the top or bottom are time intervals (see figure 11-34 for a Gantt chart template).

Each step in the project is represented by a line starting at the planned beginning date and ending at the planned completion date. The chart can show parallel activities or activities that are supposed to happen simultaneously and the relative time the various steps take. The finished Gantt chart shows the minimum time you need to complete your implementation plan, the appropriate sequence of steps, and which steps can be accomplished at the same time. User-friendly project management software exists (for example, Quickscheduler™, Harvard Project Manager™, Superproject™, and TimeLine™) that will develop Gantt charts for you. All you need to do is enter the steps in your plan and their start and end dates (see figure 11-35).

Note: To make Gantt charts even more useful, add a second line to show the real schedule as you proceed through implementation. At a glance, you can see whether you're on or off schedule by drawing a second line in another color below the original line for each step. The original line represents the plan; the second line represents the reality.

Work Sheets for Anticipating Problems

The chart in figure 11-36 (p. 183) can help you to anticipate and troubleshoot obstacles to the effective implementation of your plan and the achievement of your desired results. If you completed a force-field analysis, some of the restraining forces can be entered here.

Tree Diagrams for Action Planning

In addition to the other tools mentioned, consider using tree diagrams (tool 15) to visualize your implementation plan. Figure 11-37 (p. 184) is an example of a tree diagram used to summarize an ambitious, multipronged plan to improve employee behavior toward outpatients in a large outpatient clinic.

Storyboards

Florida Power and Light, the first Deming Award winner, presents the storyboard as an excellent way to tell a quality story and portray the plan for implementing, testing, and standardizing your improvement. As described by QUALTEC, Inc., a subsidiary of Florida Power and Light,[3] the storyboard organizes a pictorial representation of an improvement process (see figure 11-38, p. 186).

In the first frame of the QUALTEC storyboard, the team provides information about itself, often with pictures of team members and recognition of their efforts. The next seven frames tell the quality improvement story using the process QUALTEC advocates. These steps of the process correspond to the PDCA model for process improvement described earlier in this book.

Figure 11-34. Template for a Gantt Chart

Step/Task	Time Intervals: Period									
	1	2	3	4	5	6	7	8	9	10
1										
2										
3										
4										
5										
6										
7										

Figure 11-35. Example of a Simple Gantt Chart

Objective: To improve written brochures and checklists that describe discharge process to patients and physicians

Date: Week 1: Jan. 8

Action Plan

Activity	Responsibility	Time Schedule: Week													
		1	2	3	4	5	6	7	8	9	10	11	12	13	14
Collect current written materials	Pat	▬													
Convene physicians/nurses to review quality	Hal		▬												
Review with customers; pinpoint problems	Jack			▬											
Revise content	Pat/Jack					▬									
Show to customers; pilot a draft	Hal									▬					
Revise based on feedback	Pat/Jack										▬				
Physician/nurse approval	Hal											▬			
Typeset/print	Helen												▬		
Replace old version with new	Cindy														▬
Promote; send new version to nurses, physicians	Helen/Max														▬

Each step of the improvement story provides objectives, key activities, helpful tools, and checkpoints. The checkpoints help team members to focus on the necessary action-planning activities for each section as it is completed. Many teams post their storyboards so that team members can follow progress and make suggestions by attaching sticky notes to the storyboard.

One of the most important parts of the storyboard relates to future plans, referred to by Nadler and Hibino[4] as the "solution-after-next" principle. A common failing of problem solvers is not looking beyond the immediate problem and its solution to the solution after next. There is a danger of unfreezing to solve the immediate problem and refreezing at the new solution, rather than developing alternative solutions that consider future needs.

By using the storyboard to push you to foresee and consider the solution after next, you will increase the likelihood of long-term thinking and anticipating the consequences and further challenges key to holding gains over your competition and staying at the forefront.

Figure 11-36. Anticipatory Problems Work Sheet

Desired result:

Summary of strategy:

Scale:
0 = Not at all
1 = Not very
2 = Moderately
3 = Very
4 = Extremely

What Might Go Wrong	How Likely?	How Serious?	Priority	Contributory Factors or Causes	Preventive Actions	By Whom?	When?	Actions That Minimize Effects	By Whom?	When?
		×	=							
		×	=							
		×	=							
		×	=							
		×	=							
		×	=							

Reprinted, with permission, from Leebov, W., and Scott, G. *Health Care Managers in Transition: Shifting Roles and Changing Organizations.* San Francisco: Jossey-Bass, 1990.

Figure 11-37. Tree Diagram Used to Summarize an Improvement Plan

	Set clear expectations	Convene "stars" to define excellent behavior
		Write up expectations
		Get staff reactions in focus groups
		Revise; build into job descriptions
	Provide training	Identify key skills needed
		Find training resources
		Prework with supervisors
		Reserve place, dates
Improve staff behavior toward outpatients		Promote to supervisors
		Conduct sessions
		Evaluate
	Monitor	Develop/refine patient survey
		Design trend charts for wall
		Institute regular assessments
		Train data collectors/analyzers
		Run regular meetings to review results
		Feed results to teams for problem solving
	Provide supervisory coaching and support	Install expectations of supervisor as role model
		Train supervisors in customer relations
		Hold supervisor support groups for mutual helping
		Hold administrator meetings to explore barrier removal

Model for Action Planning

Following is a straightforward model for action planning that integrates the use of several of the tools of process improvement in a logical sequence:

1. Look at a flowchart of the improvement you want to implement.
2. Brainstorm steps needed to implement the improvement.
3. Cluster these steps using affinity charting.
4. Sequence the activities you generated so far by drawing a flowchart of the steps needed in your implementation plan (not in the process improvement itself).
5. Methodically go through the flowchart and list the resources needed at each step: the people whose operation, participation, and/or help you need; the supplies; the approvals; the time; and so forth. Modify the implementation flowchart to include the steps you need to go through in order to secure these resources.
6. Complete an anticipating-problems work sheet or a force-field analysis to anticipate problems or restraining forces. Revise your flowchart to incorporate actions that will prevent problems you anticipate or will minimize restraining forces.
7. Hold a focus group with the people involved in implementation. Show them the flowchart, walk through the implementation process, and ask for their help

in debugging and troubleshooting it. Revise your plans on the basis of their feedback.

8. Create a tree diagram that visually portrays your implementation plan.
9. Draw a Gantt chart that shows each activity spread over time with responsibilities assigned.
10. Develop a storyboard that tells the whole story.

References

1. King, B. *Hoshin Planning.* Methuen, MA: GOAL/QPC, 1989.

2. Nadler, G., and Hibino, S. *Breakthrough Thinking.* New York City: Prima Publishing and Communications, 1990.

3. QUALTEC. *Storyboard.* Palm Beach Gardens, FL: Florida Power and Light, 1989.

4. Nadler and Hibino.

Figure 11-38. Quality Improvement Storyboard

Team Information	1. Reason for Improvement
A Place to: • Show team name, members' pictures and names if desired. • Post Team Project Planning Worksheet. • Display team meeting minutes. • Solicit comments using self-stick notes. • Recognize individuals who provided support to the team. 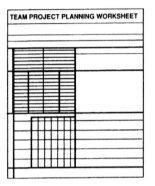 TEAM PROJECT PLANNING WORKSHEET	**Objective:** Identify a theme (problem area) and the reason for working on it. **Key Activities:** • Research for themes: —Review departmental indicators —Survey internal/external customers —Interview individuals from the work area • Consider customer needs to help select the theme. • Set indicator to track the theme. • Determine how much improvement is needed. • Show impact of the theme • Schedule the QI Story activities. • Describe the procedure used in the problem area. **Helpful Tools/Techniques:** • Graph • Process flow chart • Control chart • Control system **Checkpoints:** 1. The criteria for selection were customer oriented. 2. The indicator correctly represented the theme. 3. The need for improvement was demonstrated using data. 4. A schedule for completing the QI Story steps was developed.
4. Countermeasures	**5. Results**
Objective: Plan and implement countermeasures that will correct the root causes of the problem. **Key Activities:** • Develop and evaluate potential countermeasures which: —Attack verified root causes —Meet customer's valid requirements —Prove to be cost beneficial • Develop an action plan that: —Answers who, what, when, where & how —Reflects the barriers and aids needed for success • Obtain cooperation and approvals. • Implement countermeasures. **Helpful Tools/Techniques:** • Cost benefit analysis • Barriers and aids • Countermeasures matrix • Action plan **Checkpoints:** 13. Selected countermeasures attacked verified root causes. 14. Countermeasures were consistent with meeting customer valid requirements. 15. Countermeasures were cost beneficial. 16. Action plan answered who, what, when, where, & how. 17. Action plan reflected the barriers & aids necessary for successful implementation.	**Objective:** Confirm that the problem and its root causes have been decreased and the target for improvement has been met. **Key Activities:** • Confirm the effects of the countermeasures, checking to see if the root causes have been reduced. • Compare the problem before and after using the same indicator. • Compare the results obtained to the target. • Implement additional countermeasures, if results are not satisfactory. **Helpful Tools/Techniques:** • Histogram • Control chart • Pareto diagram • Graph **Checkpoints:** 18. Root causes have been reduced. 19. Tracking indicator was the same one used in the reason for improvement. 20. Results met or exceeded target. (If not, cause was addressed.)

2. Current Situation	3. Analysis
Objective:	**Objective:**
Select a problem and set a target for improvement.	Identify and verify the root causes of the problem.
Key Activities:	**Key Activities:**
• Collect data on all aspects of the theme. • Stratify the theme from various viewpoints. • Select a problem from the stratification of the theme. • Identify the customer's valid requirements. • Write a clear problem statement. • Utilize the data to establish the target.	• Perform cause and effect analysis on the problem. • Continue analysis to the level of actionable root causes. • Select the root causes with probable greatest impact. • Verify the selected root causes with data.
Helpful Tools/Techniques:	**Helpful Tools/Techniques:**
• Checksheet • Control chart • Histogram • Graph • Pareto diagram	• Cause & effect diagram • Histogram • Checksheet • Graph • Pareto diagram • Scatter diagram
Checkpoints:	**Checkpoints:**
5. The situation was stratified to a component level specific enough to analyze. 6. Customer valid requirements were identified. 7. Problem statement addressed the gap between the current and targeted values. 8. The methodology in establishing goals/target was identified.	9. Cause & effect analysis was performed on the problem. 10. Root causes were taken to an actionable level. 11. Root causes with probable greatest impact were selected. 12. Data was used to verify the root causes.

6. Standardization	7. Future Plans
Objective:	**Objective:**
Prevent the problem and its root causes from recurring.	Plan what to do about any remaining problems and evaluate the team's effectiveness.
Key Activities:	**Key Activities:**

• Assure that countermeasures become part of daily work:
  —Create/revise the work process
  —Create/revise standards
• Train employees on revised process and/or standards and explain need.
• Establish periodic checks with assigned responsibilities to monitor countermeasures.
• Consider areas for replication.
	• Analyze and evaluate any remaining problems
	• Plan further actions if necessary.
	• Review lessons learned related to problem solving skills and group dynamics (team effectiveness):
	  —What was done well
	  —What could be improved
	  —What could be done differently

Helpful Tools/Techniques:	**Helpful Tools/Techniques:**
• Control system • Procedure • Control chart • Training • Graph	• Action plan • P D C A
Checkpoints:	**Checkpoints:**
21. Method to assure countermeasures become part of daily work was developed (include applicable training). 22. Periodic checks were put in place with assigned responsibility to monitor the countermeasures. 23. Specific areas for replication were considered.	24. Any remaining problems of the theme will be addressed. 25. Applied PDCA to lessons learned. 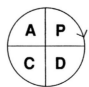

Part IV

Meeting the Quality Management Challenge

Beyond the Barriers: Toward Experimentation and Continuous Learning

I n the authors' consulting work with health care organizations on service and quality improvement, administrators have voiced several frustrations that inspired this book:

- "We feel good about what we're doing, but we lack confidence in it because we cannot measure it. Along the way, I wish we could tell how we are doing over time."
- "We have a vision and mission in place and many programs and practices that support effective management, but we do not have ways to hold our managers accountable. I wish we could somehow hold managers accountable for quality in their departments."
- "I wish every manager felt responsible for making improvements in their own departments and with other departments they are interdependent with all the time."
- "When we have launched a 'change' strategy in the past, we got started with a bang. But our middle managers watch what is happening rather than change the way they do their jobs. Somehow, managing for continuous improvement has to become inherent in the way they do their jobs. It has to become a routine, not a program or even a set of short-lived teams."
- "I wish we were more systematic in our approach. We're artistic about improving service here, but I do not think we're scientific enough."

All this points to a need to move *beyond the art* of service and quality improvement *to become scientific and methodical* in our approach to management. Unfortunately, when some people think of *the scientist,* they think of someone who collects data and "draws confusions."

The "science" we are talking about here is epitomized in the customer-driven management process presented in this book:

- Identify your customers.
- Consult with them to learn their expectations.
- Identify appropriate professional standards.
- Translate customer expectations and professional standards into operational requirements within your area of expertise.

- Create measures you can use to monitor customer satisfaction, operational performance, and professional standards.
- Use the measures you developed.
- Share the results with your staff.
- Make sense out of the results and identify improvement opportunities.
- Make process improvements.

This is a *closed-loop process*. In other words:

1. Figure out what's important.
2. Figure out how to provide it.
3. See how you're doing.
4. Work to improve it.

This process is scientific and it is common sense. Most managers would undoubtedly agree that with such a process in place, over the long haul management would be able to control quality; meet ever-rising standards; spark widespread involvement; and make concrete, tangible, and valuable improvements.

The benefits need not be belabored:

- Employees respect what management inspects.
- The ability to show results will enhance accountability for results.
- Measurement leads to control.
- Making continuous improvement a routine will encourage improvement to happen routinely.

This sounds good on paper, but how ready are you to develop yourself and your skills and to take the necessary risks with your staff, peers, and supervisors to make customer-driven management and continuous improvement your everyday way of managing?

☐ Barriers

Some people are "allergic" to numbers and are repelled by what, at first glance, looks like a numerical approach to management. However, the techniques involved in the approaches described in this book can be learned with minimum reliance on complicated formulas and theories. In our work with managers, we have witnessed some resistance to this more scientific approach to quality management, but the resistance has usually been more attitudinal than skill based. With some help, managers who decide to manage according to this back-to-basics model can and do learn the required skills.

However, resistant managers offer *six excuses* for why they cannot or do not want to follow this kind of model. As you read the following excuses, ask yourself whether you identify with any of them. If you, as a change agent, are not a believer in customer-driven management and continuous quality improvement, you will have trouble adopting the model or even helping your colleagues and organization advance in that direction.

Excuse 1: We Do This Already

This response recalls the old cartoon in which Charlie Brown and Lucy are playing baseball. The batter hits a long ball to the outfield. Charlie Brown races toward it, yelling, "I got it, I got it!" He ends up nowhere near the ball as it hits the ground and the batter circles to third base. Out of the corner of her mouth, Lucy says, "I guess 'I got it' can mean a lot of things."

Managers who look at this model and say, "Oh, sure. Of course. So what's new? I do that," are a little like Charlie Brown. They may think they're already doing it, but they are most likely "nowhere near the ball." They think, "I know my customers' needs very well because I have been catering to them for years. And I'm sure I make improvements all the time." But they are taking this for granted without looking at the situation with fresh eyes and trying new approaches to meeting customer expectations.

Excuse 2: To Measure, You Have to Oversimplify

Some think that when you focus on a select few variables, you oversimplify and thus reduce what you are measuring to absurdity. They say, "Indicators of quality miss the essence." Certainly, if you pick two indicators of quality for a particular customer group, you are missing many other important variables. But narrowing down your focus to a couple of rationally chosen indicators helps you and staff see the forest through the trees.

David Broder (a columnist for the *Washington Post*) gave a powerful speech in which he said the following:[1]

> Americans are content with the way things are but they are concerned about where we are heading. What America lacks is *a measuring stick by which we can gauge performance of those things that will determine whether we achieve our longterm goals* of making this a strong, prosperous, just, and decent society.
>
> Suppose the President were to tell his or her cabinet to come up with one or two challenges in their areas most critical for the nation's future. These challenges should be specific enough to permit measurement. The Energy Secretary might suggest that energy efficiency is an important measure of our future strength. The Labor Secretary might propose we focus on youth employment, the Commerce Secretary on gains in productivity, and the Education Secretary might suggest that reducing the school dropout rate is the most important challenge in his or her area. The Defense Secretary might use the percentage of high school . . . graduates as a way of measuring readiness.
>
> We could soon have a yardstick of national performance visible in chart form in every classroom, factory, office, bank, city hall, and hospital across the land — a daily reminder of the challenges we face as a people. You know that Americans are both community-minded and competitive enough that these national challenges would quickly become individual goals we would stretch to attain.

Neither David Broder nor any American would say that what we chose to measure is *all* that is important to us. But it certainly would be powerful to keep our eyes on those goals and our progressive steps toward achieving them.

It is equally important for health care organizations, albeit on a smaller scale. We need to select the attributes of quality that are powerful satisfiers for our customers, create our own yardsticks, and use measurement to keep our own and our staff's eyes on the goal and how we're doing. Because our employees are caring people with a competitive spirit, these quality challenges would quickly become individual goals we would stretch to attain.

Excuse 3: I Don't Have Time

Absolutely true. It is the rare health care manager who is not running ragged in today's environment, who does not have very lean or inadequate staffing and many daily fires to put out. But let us not confuse "busy-ness" with results. If a manager has no means of tracking department performance, he or she may pour energy into working very hard at what might be the wrong things. Quality means *doing the right things right* in order to meet customer expectations. Unfortunately, many managers work very hard *doing the* wrong things day in and day out. If you implement the kind of customer-driven management process described in the preceding chapters, you will know when you are not meeting customer expectations and will have a mechanism for determining root causes of problems that, when tackled, will enable you to spend your valuable time doing the right things.

When people cite the all-purpose excuse "I don't have time," it brings to mind an astute old adage that is helpful to remember in these turbulent times: "It's better to wear out than to rust out."

Excuse 4: I Can't Do Anything about It Anyway; I Don't Have the Power to Make the Changes Needed to Improve Performance

It's a new day. Administrators want their organizations to excel on quality dimensions, which means they are increasingly willing to support managers engaged in the quest for continuous improvement. It is time to question frustrations of the past and take personal responsibility for working harder and asserting ourselves more than ever to push the bureaucracy and confront administrators who we perceive are blocking our efforts to improve quality.

We need a new feistiness and persistence to see what we can accomplish if, within our own realms of influence, we engage our employees in ongoing improvement. A tremendous amount can be done within our ranks. If you do not believe this, go into any department in your organization and conduct a meeting with that department's staff that goes something like this: "You have 20 minutes. In small groups, come up with *any improvement* we can make to increase our customers' satisfaction. The rules are as follows: It cannot cost anything, and it has to be 100 percent within our power to implement, without anyone else's cooperation or approval." We guarantee you will see improvements.

We have to rekindle our belief that we can spark change, take responsibility for making change happen, and stop finger-pointing as a convenient excuse for making tomorrow an extension of yesterday instead of the new day and the new experiment it needs to be. And when we hit barriers beyond our control, we need to attack them by asking the executives who lead us for their conviction, skills, and resources.

Excuse 5: I Don't Think I Know How

Many managers resist change because of a deep and often embarrassing feeling of inadequacy. They might think to themselves, "I don't know how to do this. I never did it before, and I'm scared that others will see my incompetence. If people see me as incompetent, I might lose my job."

Fears about inadequacy deserve questioning. Finally, after years of standards, norms, and expectations, we are talking about *continuous* improvement; that concept applies as much to you, the manager, as it does to your organization. If you need time to equip yourself with an expanded repertoire of quality management practices, so be it. Join the crowd as we all learn and fine-tune our skills. Our industry is not filled with experts at systematic approaches to continuous improvement. We have not needed these skills before, but we do now. So let's learn them.

Fears about job insecurity are very real; middle-manager ranks are decreasing. It's called *flattening the organization* and *streamlining*. But this is being done not because managers are struggling to improve quality and customer satisfaction, but because those managers in question are *not* doing anything different today than they did yesterday— and maintaining the status quo is not the job any longer. A surge in new learning and risk taking is essential. As one CEO said, "If my managers aren't fired with enthusiasm for quality improvement, they will be fired with enthusiasm."

Excuse 6: This Isn't Fun

For many people, especially those uncomfortable with *methodical* approaches to quality improvement, it may not look like fun. As one manager said, "I need this like a giraffe needs strep throat!" Although start-up can certainly be tedious, once you decide to implement this kind of model, it is indeed fun and even revitalizing. People become excited with the experiment, the challenge of competing against past performance to achieve new heights.

☐ Beyond the Barriers

These and other forms of resistance are deeply felt. The question remains: What can you do to manage for continuous improvement? In this book, we have suggested implementing quality management in all its dimensions as the regular routine in your department. This entails installing customer-driven management, which, according to our model, means identifying your customers' expectations, designing your services to meet those expectations, measuring satisfaction and operational performance, and using the results to identify and pursue improvement opportunities continuously and relentlessly.

It also involves embracing the managerial mind-set or attitudes that drive your standards ever upward and spark your initiative, experimentation, and sense of responsibility. The results will be heightened customer and staff satisfaction; streamlined, seamless service delivery; financial viability for your organization; and revitalization and renewal for you in your role as a manager.

Take a long, hard look at your own resistance. Find a way to make yourself comfortable, even if it is not your style. And build your own skills:

- If you feel insecure using a scientific approach, admit it. Make it okay for others to admit it, too.
- Get help. Learn! Read. Experiment. Try new ways.

As a manager in your organization, you are in a pivotal position to make change and spark continuous quality improvement. Use that power as a change agent to make your people, your organization, and yourself continuous learners for the sake of ever-better quality, heightened customer satisfaction, and personal renewal.

Reference

1. Broder, D. *Washington Post.* 1988.

Chapter 13

Case Study: The PDCA Model in Practice

This chapter describes one process improvement initiative implemented by the Quality First Discharge Team at Holston Valley Hospital and Medical Center in Kingsport, Tennessee, and the figures reproduced here are used with their permission. Both the planning and implementation of the improvement are described. As you will see, for the most part the steps fall into the four phases of the plan–do–check–act (PDCA) model described in chapter 8.

☐ Step 1: The Hospital's Administration Identified the Problem

The hospital conducted focus groups with patients and their family members in an attempt to identify the attributes of quality that these customers use to evaluate their hospital stay. "Promptness of discharge" was one of several attributes identified as very important to patients and their families.

The hospital then instituted a patient survey that polled satisfaction with attributes of hospitalization important to its customers. The hospital distributed the survey to all discharged patients and tallied the results monthly. After three months, it became clear that many patients were dissatisfied with the organization's performance on "promptness of discharge," as shown in figure 13-1. During this three-month period, an average of 35 percent of the patients who responded to the survey gave discharge promptness a rating of fair or poor.

As a result, hospital leaders targeted discharge delays as an important improvement opportunity and chartered an improvement team to work on reducing those delays. The team consisted of those people most closely involved in the discharge process, including representatives of nursing, transport services, and billing.

☐ Step 2: Suppliers, Inputs, Outputs, Customers, and Customer Expectations Regarding the Discharge Process Were Identified

In discussions with the parties involved, the team identified the suppliers, inputs, process, outputs, and customers of the discharge process, as follows:

Figure 13-1. Trend Chart: Patient Dissatisfaction with Promptness of Discharge

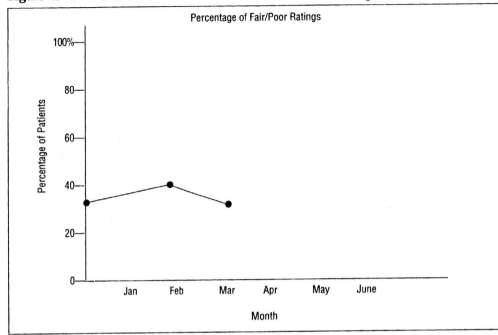

- Suppliers: physicians
- Inputs: discharge orders
- Process: discharge process
- Outputs: patients
- Customers: patients' families and/or friends

The team already knew that patients and their families felt delays were too long. To find out what they meant by "too long," team members telephoned a sample of former patients and asked them. Most patients said, "Once I'm told I can leave, I want to get moving and get out! That means not waiting for people—not waiting for help getting me ready, not waiting for someone to pick me up, not waiting in your billing office—not waiting." The team concluded that patients would tolerate *time well spent*, but not time lags in which no progress was made toward their departure.

☐ Step 3: The Current Discharge Process Was Flowcharted

The team then mapped out the current discharge process on a "block" flowchart that clearly showed not only the steps in the process, but also who was responsible for each step, for example, nursing, transportation services, patient accounts (see figure 13-2). In this case, the purpose of flowcharting was to develop a shared understanding of the current process and to figure out which data should be collected to understand the steps that most contributed to discharge delays.

☐ Step 4: Data Were Collected

The team collected baseline data. The actual discharge time for 31 patients was charted over a two-week period (see figure 13-3, p. 200). Then, to find out *where* the delays were occur-

Figure 13-2. Flowchart for the Current Discharge Process

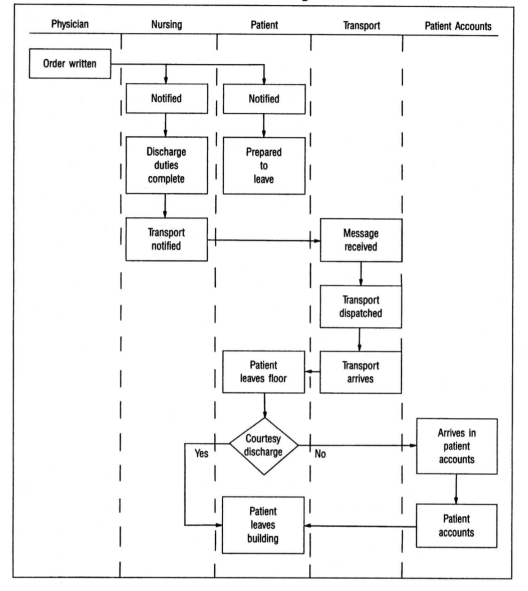

ring and *how long* they were, the team collected data about the length of time consumed at each step in the process under both ideal and real conditions. They asked:

- Under *ideal* conditions, that is, assuming there were no delays and that all staff involved performed well, how long would it take to complete each step? For example:
  - From the time the physician writes the discharge order to the time the patient is notified
  - From the time the nurse is notified to the time he or she completes discharge duties
  - From the time transport is notified to the time a transporter is dispatched
  - From the time the transporter arrives in the patient's room to the time the transporter and patient depart
  - From the time the transporter and patient arrive in patient accounts to the time they leave

Figure 13-3. Run Chart of Discharge Time

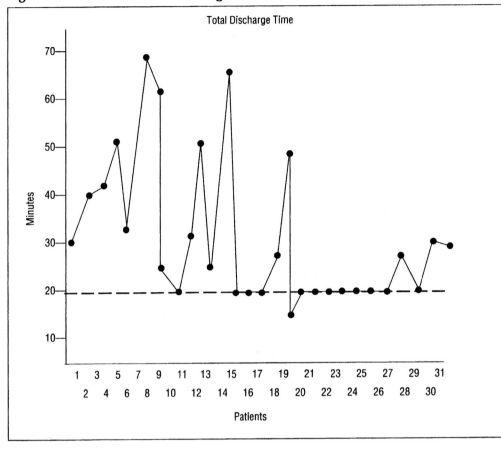

—From the time they leave patient accounts to the time the patient arrives at the exit

The team determined this ideal or "target time" by consulting (and sometimes timing with a stopwatch) the people who do the work to find out how long it actually takes to do each step (time on task) under ideal conditions.

• Under *real* conditions, how long does it take to complete each step? The team developed simple *time logs* to enable people involved in the process to record times over a two-week period (see figure 13-4). Team members divided responsibility for training the people in the best position to log times for their piece of the process.

☐ Step 5: The Data Were Summarized and the Delays Identified

The team synthesized the data from the various time logs. The ideal time was compared to the actual time involved at each step to determine the steps where the biggest delays occurred (see figure 13-5).

The team then asked whether there were a select few steps in the process where the longest time lags occurred. Using a Pareto chart (see figure 13-6, p. 202), team members found that the steps involving transport and patient accounts were responsible for a disproportionate share of the delays. To use their time wisely, team members decided to target these steps because improvements here would have a greater effect on reducing delays than all the other steps combined.

Figure 13-4. Time Logs

To record time made aware of signed discharge order (completed by nurses):

	Patient's Name	Room	Time
1.	Smith	203	11:20
2.	Harding	208	1:30
3.	Marcus	212	1:52

To measure the time lag between receiving the transport request and dispatching the transporter, the receptionist in transport completed this log:

	Patient's Name	Time I Received Call for Transport	Time Transporter Was Dispatched
1	Smith	11:40	11:55
2	Harding	1:55	2:30
3	Marcus	2:45	3:30
4	Overson	2:50	3:40
5	Tulley	3:05	4:00
6	Johnson	3:20	4:15

To measure the time lags between arrival in the patient's room, arrival at patient accounts, and departure from hospital exit, transporters recorded arrival times on this log:

	Patient's Name	In Patient's Room	Patient Accounts	Exit Door
1	Smith	12:00	12:10	12:35
2	Harding	2:40	2:55	3:25
3	Marcus	3:45	4:10	4:45
4	Overson	3:50	4:20	4:50
5	Tulley	4:15	4:40	5:10
6	Johnson	4:30	4:35	5:30

Figure 13-5. Chart Showing Delays in the Process of Patient Discharge

Process Step	Average Times (in minutes)		
	Actual Time	− Ideal Time	= Time Lag
From time physician writes order to time patient notified	20	5	15
From time nurse is notified to time nurse completes discharge duties	35	15	20
From time transport is notified to dispatch	38	5	33
From time transport arrives in patient's room to time transport departs with patient	10	3	7
From arrival in Patient Accounts to departure	45	5	40
From time they leave Patient Accounts to time patient arrives at exit	10	5	5

Figure 13-6. Pareto Chart of Delays in the Process of Patient Discharge, in Descending Order

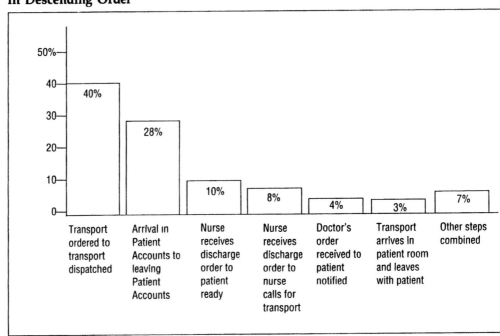

☐ Step 6: Root Causes of Delays in Patient Accounts Were Sought

The team used brainstorming and cause-and-effect diagrams to hunt for the root causes of the delays in patient accounts.

Brainstorming

First, the team brainstormed their theories about possible causes and came up with the following responses:

- Department understaffed
- All patients go there but shouldn't
- Computer problems
- Patients weren't prepared to bring necessary information
- Patients not well, hard to concentrate
- Patients angry at having to talk money at end of stay
- Staff inadequately trained
- Not enough information collected earlier
- Lost preadmission information
- Patients in bathroom when it's their turn and the bathroom is far away
- Need to hunt for lost charges

Cause-and-Effect Diagram

To complement their list of causes, two team members conducted a focus group with patient accounts staff to find out their theories on the subject. They used a cause-and-effect diagram to help focus group members consider factors related to equipment, methods, patients, and staff (see figure 13-7).

Figure 13-7. Cause-and-Effect Diagram

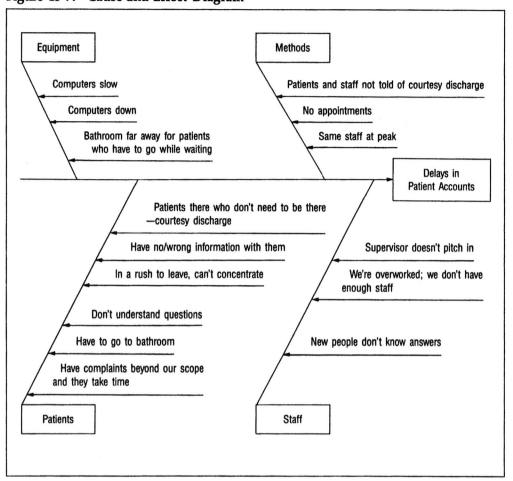

☐ Step 7: The Team Voted to Choose the "Big Two" Causes

The facilitator asked patient accounts staff to look at the many causes generated and, drawing on their firsthand experience, to vote for the "big two." The following two received the highest number of votes:

- Patients are in patient accounts who do not need to be there.
- Patient accounts is understaffed for the number of patients it has to see.

☐ Step 8: Root Causes of the Causes Were Sought

Because money was tight and the team felt that understaffing is often a smoke screen for inefficiencies in a process, the facilitator asked staff to do a quick tree diagram (the why–why form) to dig deeper into the root causes of the causes already identified. As can be seen from figure 13-8, every cause was broken down into at least two more specific causes.

☐ Step 9: Discussion Was Used to Select the Primary Root Cause

The improvement team met to discuss the results of their hunt for root causes and focused on the following as the primary cause of delays in patient accounts:

Figure 13-8. Why–Why Tree Diagram

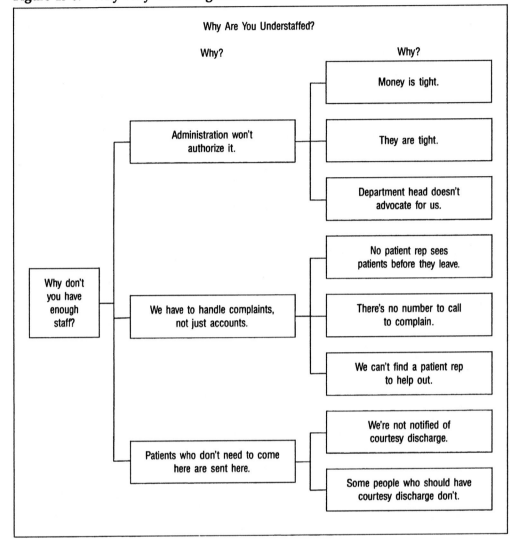

- Patient accounts is overloaded and keeps people waiting because patients come there who don't need to.
- The patients who don't need to come there are those with courtesy discharge status.
- The problem is that in some cases, neither the patient nor the transporter knows of the courtesy discharge status, and so they come to patient accounts needlessly, wait unnecessarily, and clog the department's work load.

☐ Step 10: Brainstorming Was Used to Generate Improvements Related to the Root Cause

The root cause was summarized as follows: Many people qualified for courtesy discharge status came to patient accounts even though it was unnecessary. Team members brainstormed alternative solutions or countermeasures to this problem and arrived at two:

- Fix the system so that courtesy discharge status is known to all key parties.
  - Patients should know so that they can provide a check on the transporter and people in patient accounts.

-The nursing unit should know so that the nurses can tell the transport office where the transporter should take the patient.
-The transporter should know so that he or she will know whether to take the patient to the door or to patient accounts.
-Patient accounts should know so that in case patients arrive who do not need to be there, the department can immediately help them leave without making them wait their turn.

- Look into whether more patients can be granted courtesy discharge status without significantly reducing uncollectible accounts. This would make more patients happier, ease the clog in patient accounts, and reduce the demand for transporter time (the source of the second-longest delays).

☐ Step 11: The Team Planned Their Improvements

Team members then asked themselves two simple questions:

- How can we clean up the courtesy discharge process?
- Can we get courtesy discharges for more patients, because it would save patient transport and patient accounts staff time?

They talked with knowledgeable people about the relevant steps of the process and quickly determined how to improve the process related to courtesy discharges. They decided to make the following changes:

- Add a field to the patient's computer screen indicating "COURTESY DISCHARGE   YES/NO."
- When nurses call in a transport request, they will specify a courtesy discharge or not so that the transporter will know whether to bypass patient accounts.

These changes were summarized on the flowchart shown in figure 13-9.

☐ Step 12: The Changes Were Implemented on a Trial Basis and Tracked for Results

A field was added to the patients' computer screen indicating their discharge status, and nursing agreed to inform the transport service of the same. To see whether these changes actually worked to reduce delays in patient accounts, the team logged the overall length of the discharge process to see whether it decreased significantly. For a trial run of a month, they also had patient accounts staff log patient time to see whether their remaining patients experienced reduced waiting times. The information showed that waiting times in patient accounts were reduced by 35 percent.

☐ Step 13: The Results Were Evaluated

The results were a dramatic reduction in discharge time for people who bypassed patient accounts and, therefore, a positive impact on the overall discharge time. Figure 13-10 shows the new results of the patient survey question that originally triggered the focus on discharge delays. After solutions were instituted, negative ratings were reduced from 35 percent initially to 18 percent.

Figure 13-9. Flowchart Showing Process Change

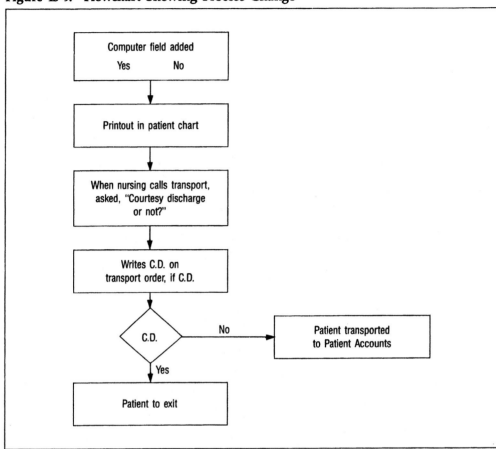

Figure 13-10. Trend Chart of Patient Dissatisfaction with Promptness of Discharge

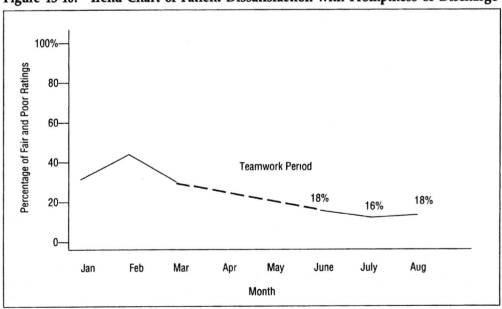

☐ Step 14: The Team Decided to Experiment Further with Reducing Delays

In an effort to reduce delays even further and thus increase patient satisfaction even more, the team decided to propose two experiments to the hospital administration:

- *Liberalize eligibility for courtesy discharge and study the effects.* Given that courtesy discharge status dramatically reduced departure time for patients, the team wondered why more patients did not receive this status, that is, what the effect would be if the hospital liberalized the policy determining eligibility for courtesy discharge by offering it to people with only partial insurance. Would a higher percentage of accounts cause collection problems? If not, granting more patients courtesy discharge status would free up transport hours and patient accounts time and would produce happier patients.
- *Bedside service from patient accounts.* Team members also wondered whether it would be possible for patient accounts staff to go to the patient, especially during the busiest discharge hours, when transport delays were greatest. That is, what if a few patient accounts staff members would go to patients' rooms instead of requiring transporters to bring the patients to them?

The team decided to propose the testing on a trial basis of a liberalized policy for granting courtesy discharge status to patients. They also began investigating a system of roving account reps.

☐ Step 15: The Team Standardized the Change

The essence of the changes instituted to better designate patients with courtesy discharge were the following: addition of a computer field for designating courtesy discharge status, filled in by admissions; a line designating that status printed on the patient's chart; nursing unit secretaries alerted to this line when ordering transport for a patient ready to leave; and transport informed that courtesy discharge patients were to be taken to the exit and not to patient accounts.

To ensure conformance with these changes, the team set up orientation sessions with:

- Supervisors in admissions, who needed to be sure that the computer field on courtesy discharge status was filled in
- Supervisors in nursing, who were responsible for ensuring that unit secretaries knew how to read the courtesy discharge field on the chart and how to order transport for discharged patients when the field said yes
- Dispatchers in transport services, who needed to ensure that transporters knew whether to take patients to patient accounts or to the exit

The supervisors then trained their staff. And, finally, members of the improvement team did monthly spot checks for three months to ensure conformance. Specifically, they did retrospective analyses of patients' charts that had arrived in nursing to see the percentage of charts for which the courtesy discharge field had been filled in. They also analyzed the log kept by the dispatcher in transport to see the percentage of times the medical secretaries appropriately notified transport of courtesy discharge status at the time of the transport request. These efforts helped to ensure that the changes were not just designed, but were operationally implemented and instituted into the regular routine.

☐ Step 16: Monitoring Was Instituted to Hold the Gains

To monitor the process changes and hold the gains, the team saw to it that data about discharge time and patient survey results continued to be collected periodically and summarized on trend charts like those shown in figures 13-3 and 13-10.

☐ Step 17: The Team Shifted Its Attention to Delays in Transport

Although the team felt that transport time would be in greater supply now that transporters did not have to waste their time sitting in patient accounts with patients who were not supposed to be there, the team decided to touch base with people in transport services to see whether they could think of other ways to reduce delays in transport during discharge.

☐ Step 18: A Focus Group with Transporters Was Convened

The questions asked were: "Why are there delays? What can we do about them?"

The answer to the first question was simply: "We don't have enough people." The answer to the second question was: "We wouldn't need so many people if we didn't have a policy that requires us to escort *every* patient to the door."

Transporters claimed that many patients became angry because their family members were there to help them, but "hospital policy prevents patients from leaving on their own." Apparently, many patients were ambulatory and wanted to leave when they were ready. Transporters assumed the policy could not be changed.

☐ Step 19: Theory Was Investigated and Tradition Was Questioned

At its next meeting, the team asked, "How many patients could leave on their own if we allowed them to?" To check this out quickly, team members asked nurses to record whether each discharged patient needed a wheelchair or could walk out with the proper support. They charted the results for a day, believing that the percentages would not vary much from day to day. The results were interesting. They found that almost half of their patients were ambulatory and could have left on their own if the hospital had permitted it (see figure 13-11).

The team then asked, "Is there a law that every patient must be escorted to the door? If not, why are we doing it? It is obviously not making some of our patients very happy." Because no one knew the answer, team members visited the hospital's legal department and asked for a review of the policy. The question being considered was, "*Must* we transport discharged patients to the door or can we let them go on their own steam?" The legal department's answer was, "The only reason we do it this way is because we always have. It seems like the right thing to do. But, the fact is, under Tennessee law, we are not required to escort patients who prefer that we don't."

☐ Step 20: The Improvement Was Proposed and Tested

After the team and the hospital attorney reviewed the liability issues involved and determined that they were insignificant, the team proposed to hospital administration the idea of, for a trial period, giving patients their choice of leaving with an escort or leaving on their own. The administrative team agreed. The team inserted a "decision" point in their flowchart at which the nurse would ask the patient and family, "I'm planning to request that one of our transporters escort you to the door, unless you prefer leaving without help. What do you prefer?"

Figure 13-11. Pareto Chart Showing Method of Discharge, 11/10/89

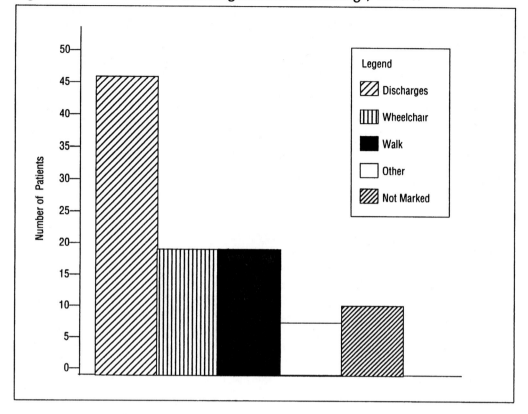

☐ Step 21: Results Were Tracked and Conclusions Drawn

Nurses recorded the number of patients who chose transport assistance and those who did not. The results were as follows: 37 percent of the patients (ambulatory walkouts) chose to leave on their own and were delighted to do so because that meant they could leave sooner. This, in turn, greatly relieved the burden on the overloaded transport service because it then had to fulfill substantially fewer dispatch orders related to discharge.

☐ Step 22: The Team Standardized the Changes

After a successful trial run, the team redrafted the flowchart to reflect the changes in patient flow during the discharge process. Because representatives of the key departments were on the team, these people immediately proceeded to integrate the changes into everyday operations (see figure 13-12).

☐ It Took All That Work to Do So Little?

With many improvements, hindsight is 20/20. You might read through this case and wonder why they didn't consider addressing the courtesy discharge status sooner. It seems so obvious. Or why hadn't the transport service or nursing department questioned the long-standing practice of escorting all patients to the door when they knew that this practice was frustrating patients. However, the fact is that most of us do what we've always done. And the systems in which we work seem to have an immune reaction in the face of suggested change. By going through a methodical process, such as PDCA, we get unstuck from our old ways, we devote team energy to new and better possibilities, and we build confidence that our suggestions for improvement will reap benefits for our customers, ourselves, and, therefore, the organization.

It can be a tedious process. The road to process improvement tends to wind and curve, with occasional obstacles and detours. Even experts in the technology of process

Figure 13-12. Revised Flowchart Standardizing Changes

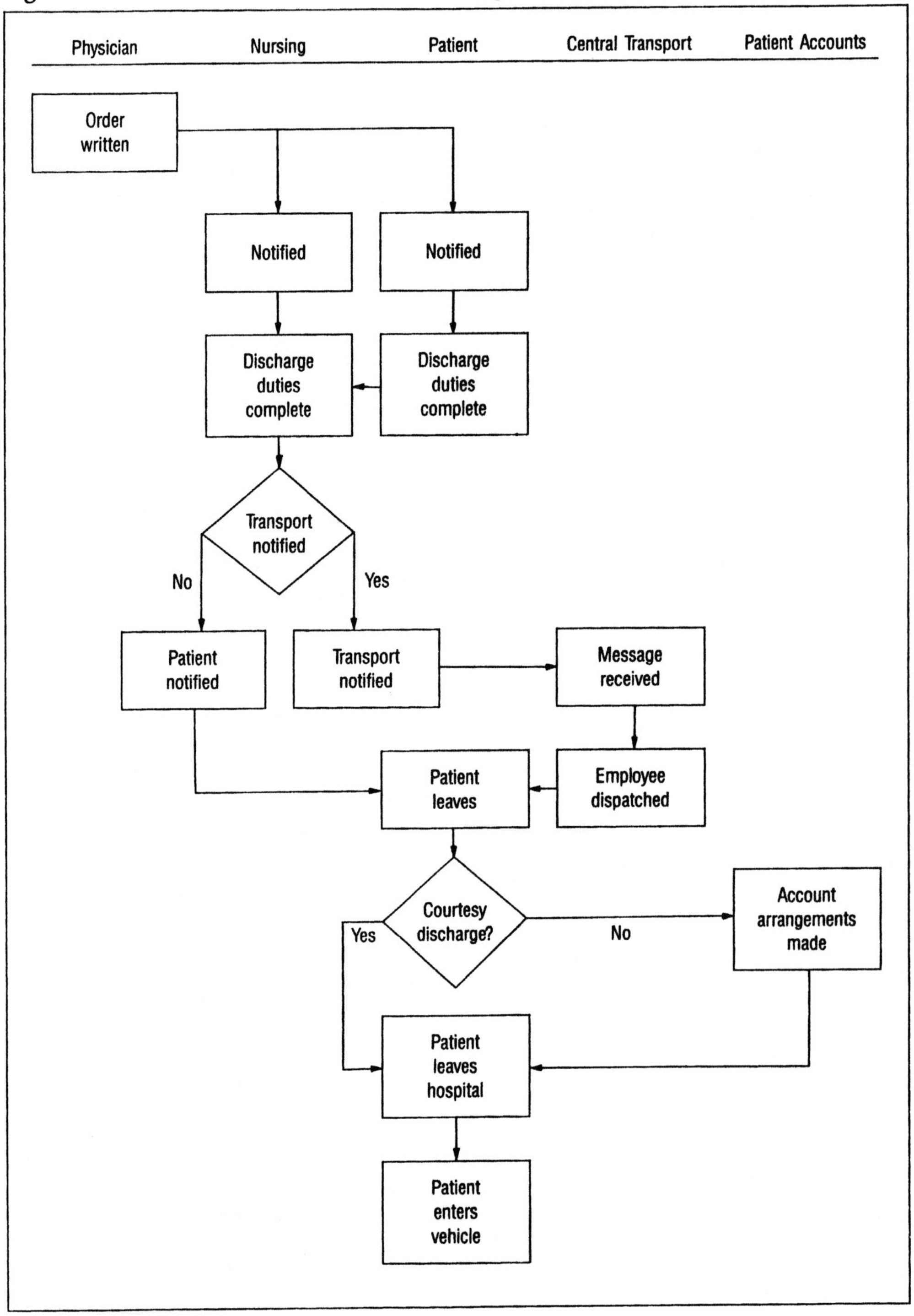

improvement find it necessary to do some meandering through the process because you cannot be sure a tool will enlighten your decision making until you try it. Sometimes it will help you, and sometimes it will not.

For that reason, you need an experimenter mind-set. You need to follow your hunch that a tool might help and then try it. If it helps, great! If it doesn't, ask yourself, "What else might help?" And you move on and try that. It takes practice and experience to become skilled not only in using the tools but also in knowing which ones to use and when.

Appendix

Resources for Continuous Improvement

Books

Asaka, T., and Ozeki, K., editors. *Handbook of Quality Tools.* Cambridge, MA: Productivity Press, 1990.

Crosby, P. *Quality Is Free: The Art of Making Quality Certain.* New York City: New American Library, 1979.

GOAL/QPC. *The Memory Jogger: A Pocket Guide of Tools for Continuous Improvement.* Methuen, MA: GOAL/QPC, 1988.

GOAL/QPC. *Memory Jogger Plus.* Methuen, MA: GOAL/QPC, 1989.

Imai, M. *Kaizen: The Key to Japan's Competitive Success.* New York City: Random House, 1986.

Juran, J. M. *Juran on Planning for Quality.* New York City: The Free Press, 1988.

King, B. *Hoshin Planning: The Developmental Approach.* Methuen, MA: GOAL/QPC, 1989.

Leebov, W. *Service Excellence: The Customer Relations Strategy for Health Care.* Chicago: American Hospital Publishing, 1988.

Leebov, W., and Scott, G. *Health Care Managers in Transition: Shifting Roles and Changing Organizations.* San Francisco: Jossey-Bass, 1990.

Nadler, G., and Hibino, S. *Breakthrough Thinking.* Rocklin, CA: Prima Publishing and Communications, 1990.

Psarouthakis, J. *Better Makes Us Best.* Cambridge, MA: Productivity Press, 1989.

Rosander, A. C. *The Quest for Quality in Services.* Milwaukee: Quality Press, American Society for Quality Control, 1989.

Scholtes, P. R., and others. *The Team Handbook.* Madison, WI: Joiner Associates, 1988.

Shewhart, W. *Economic Control of Quality of Manufactured Product.* New York City: Van Nostrand, 1931.

Shigeru, M. *Management for Quality Improvement.* Cambridge, MA: Productivity Press, 1989.

Steiber, S., and Krowinski, W. *Measuring and Managing Patient Satisfaction.* Chicago: American Hospital Publishing, 1990.

Walton, M. *The Deming Management Method.* New York City: Dodd, Mead and Co., 1986.

Newsletters/Periodicals

The Quality Letter for Healthcare Leaders
Bader & Associates
P.O. Box 2106
Rockville, MD 20847-2106
301/468-1610

Quality Progress
American Society for Quality Control
230 West Wells Street, Suite 700
Milwaukee, WI 53203
414/272-8575

Service Excellence in Practice
The Einstein Consulting Group
York and Tabor Roads
Philadelphia, PA 19141
215/456-7065

TEI: Total Employee Involvement
Productivity Press
Cambridge, MA
800/888-6485

Total Quality Newsletter
Lakewood Publications
50 South Ninth Street
Minneapolis, MN 55402
800/328-4329

Organizations/Sources of Information

American Society for Quality Control (ASQC)
230 West Wells Street
Milwaukee, WI 53203
414/272-8575

Association for Quality and Participation (AQP)
801B West Eighth Street, Suite 301
Cincinnati, OH 45203
513/381-1959

FPL QUALTEC, Inc.
P.O. Box 30459
Palm Beach Gardens, FL 33408
407/775-8300

Goal/QPC
13 Branch Street
Methuen, MA 01844
508/685-3900

Healthcare Forum
Association of Western Hospitals
830 Market Street
San Francisco, CA 94102
415/421-8810

Joint Commission on Accreditation of Healthcare Organizations
One Renaissance Boulevard
Oakbrook Terrace, IL 60161
708/916-5600

Juran Institute
88 Danbury Road
Wilton, CT 06897
203/834-1700

National Demonstration Project on Quality Improvement in Health Care
Harvard Community Health Plan
10 Brookline Place West
Brookline, MA 02146
617/730-4770

Productivity
P.O. Box 3007
Cambridge, MA 02140
800/888-6485

0-595-28366-7

Printed in the United States
40007LVS00004B/23